Children and Marital Conflict

Children and Marital Conflict

The Impact of Family Dispute and Resolution

E. MARK CUMMINGS
PATRICK DAVIES

Foreword by ROBERT E. EMERY

THE GUILFORD PRESS
New York   London

© 1994 The Guilford Press
A Division of Guilford Publications, Inc.
72 Spring Street, New York, NY 10012

Printed in the United States of America

This book is printed on acid-free paper.

Last digit is print number: 9   8   7   6   5   4   3

Library of Congress Cataloging in Publication Data
Cummings, E. Mark.
    Children and marital conflict : the impact of family dispute
and resolution / E. Mark Cummings, Patrick Davies.
        p.   cm. — (The Guilford series on social and emotional
development)
    ISBN 0-89862-304-9 (hard)—ISBN 0-89862-303-0 (pbk)
    1. Child development. 2. Family—Psychological aspects.
3. Interpersonal conflict. 4. Conflict management. I.   Davies,
Patrick. II.   Title. III.   Series.
HQ772.5.C86   1994
305.23′1—dc20   93-43572
                                                          CIP

Foreword

Mark Cummings and Patrick Davies's superb book integrates evidence from a wide array of investigations of children and marital conflict. They carefully guide the reader through this maze of studies, and the result is a volume that is at once authoritative, readable, and practical. The book constantly highlights the theme that children can be the real losers in marital disputes, yet they note that marital conflict cannot be "cured" by the best of intentions—or by divorce. Parents will fight, and, one way or another, children will encounter these disputes. But Cummings and Davies are optimists. They suggest that well-managed marital disputes can lead to outcomes that are *not* invariably negative. In fact, Cummings and Davies argue that conflict sometimes may have positive consequences.

Cummings and Davies's detailed review of this optimistic possibility reminds me why I routinely put myself in a situation that makes many people shudder. I sit down with parents who are in the middle of an acrimonious custody dispute and try to help them come to an agreement about rearing their children after divorce. Why do I do this? Why do more and more divorcing parents attempt to mediate their custody disputes? Because mismanaged conflict between parents harms children, as Cummings and Davies document with evidence from study after study. These are grown-up disputes between adults. There has to be a better way of handling them.

The authors quickly remind us that, despite the substantial body of research on negative outcomes, conflict is not inherently "bad." Obviously, parents in the middle of a divorce have many real and legitimate disputes, as do husbands and wives in their day-to-day lives. Conflict in families is inevitable, and fighting often is adaptive. Problems cannot be resolved without conflict, so the goal is not to avoid fighting. Rather, the goal is to fight constructively.

Until the last decade or two, psychologists have not focused much of their research on marital conflict. Marriage was not viewed as a fit topic for study in a discipline that focused on the individual. The neglect of relationships has begun to be reversed, however, and psychologists have investigated marital and family relationships with increasing vigor. Cummings and Davies reap evidence from this body of literature in order to document patterns of destructive conflict and to suggest how marriage partners can learn to fight in a way that protects their children and themselves.

The heart of this book focuses on a detailed consideration of marital conflict and children's well-being. Cummings is an important and influential contributor to this body of research. He has developed a simple and powerful research paradigm. He exposes children to simulated arguments between adults and systematically studies how children respond to this "background anger." In some of his studies, the background anger involves a live, "spontaneous" fight between two actors who are unknown to the children. In many studies, the children see a videotape of two actors fighting with one another, a procedure which offers both lower cost and greater experimental control. In one of my favorite paradigms, children see their mothers "fighting" over the telephone, as they simulate an argument into a dead handset.

What has Cummings found in his research? In my opinion, his most important finding is the most simple one. Children react to the fighting even though it does not concern or involve them directly. This finding is important to the wider body of research on children and marital conflict that Cummings and Davies review with care in this volume. Cummings' experiments unequivocally document that conflict can *cause*

distress among children. The effects of conflict are not mediated solely through parenting, depression, or other factors
that are correlated with marital conflict in the real world. However, Cummings and Davies do discuss how other research
indicates that marital conflict does adversely affect children, in
part, because it undermines parenting practices and each partner's feelings of self-worth.

An extremely important contribution of research on children's coping with marital conflict is that it challenges traditional psychological theories. Most of our major psychological
theories do not offer an explanation for why children should
be upset by conflict between other people. These theories focus on the individual or the dyad, but the family interactions
discussed by Cummings and Davies are triadic processes. This
work forces us to view children as being a part of a larger
system of relationships and to recognize that the quality of
these relationships affects children's individual well-being.

All marital disputes affect children, but children react in
interesting and different ways to the conflict and anger they
observe. Although some children become more aggressive
with peers after observing the fights, others (as young as one
year old) become emotionally upset in reaction to conflict. Still
other children intervene in the disputes, or at least they report
that they would like to intervene. In my view, what we are
witnessing is children's attempts at emotional regulation, a
theoretically rich and complex process. Conflict distresses children even though the dispute is not directed toward them. It
makes them mad, sad, or scared. As a result, they attempt to
regulate their own affect by intervening in the fighting. Emotions serve interpersonal functions, and interpersonal responses help the children to regulate their emotions.

Parents, therapists, and social scientists need to attend to
children's affective reactions to conflict even when the reactions are not obvious. Many children are quiet, helpful mediators. These children take too much responsibility for manag-
ing their parents' relationship, and too many parents allow (or
encourage) children to play this mediator role. I suspect that

children who have been mediators become adults who remain overly responsible in relationships. They are "enablers" who subjugate their own feelings in the service of the feelings of other people.

Whether the goal is to alter such long-term outcomes or to change more immediate ones, an extremely important— and optimistic—message of this book is that children's reactions to conflict are substantially influenced by *how* adults fight with each other. Children are more distressed by conflict that is angry or physical, an outcome that is of obvious importance. What is less obvious about children's reactions to conflict, however, is that these responses are greatly affected by whether or not the fight is resolved.

Actually, I think that "managed" is a better word than resolved because negotiating conflict is an ongoing process. As the book highlights, conflicts are not just resolved or unresolved. There are degrees to the resolution of conflict. The term management conveys this central idea. Dealing with conflict is a continuous task, not a dicotomous one. In fact, it is my view that many, perhaps most, conflicts remain unresolved in marital and family relationships. In order to get along, perhaps family members sometimes need to agree how they will disagree.

Some degree of resolution is important because, as Cummings and Davies document, children are considerably less distressed by conflict when it is resolved, even if the resolution is not complete. I suspect that when adults resolve or partially resolve their conflicts, perhaps the central message for children is *not* that the conflict has "gone away"; rather, the more important message may be that the adults will manage their conflicts themselves. In any case, the concern for parents is to attempt to reach some resolution. And if parents do manage their conflicts well, children can, in fact, learn positive lessons from seeing their parents deal effectively with disputes.

The idea that parents can—and should—manage their conflicts in order to protect and promote children's well-being is the central message of this book. For researchers, the book

offers a state-of-the-art review of the literature and a thought-
ful consideration of methodological detail. For therapists and
policy makers, the evidence offers strong support for the goal
of designing and implementing family interventions to contain
conflict. Therapists also will be able to draw much from the
practical implications of the research findings, as will parents
themselves. I have long felt that, rather than leaving the task
to professional writers, scientists should translate their research into a language understood by the public. Cummings
and Davies do not oversimplify research in this volume, but
they have taken great pains to present a complex body of
evidence in a manner that is accessible to lay as well as professional audiences.

ROBERT E. EMERY
University of Virginia

Preface

Adults marry because they hope marriage will provide happiness. Parents bring children into the world to fulfill their dreams of family, and they wish only the best for their children. The goals of marriage and having children are idealistic and positive in all but rare instances.

These points bear repeating in light of the considerable evidence of distress within the American family. Marital discord is a common occurence in families, with direct consequences for the children. In 1984, because of divorce or separation, over 9 million minors were living in one-parent families (U. S. Bureau of the Census, 1985), and 20% or more of intact marriages were "distressed."

Why this sharp contrast between intentions and outcomes within the American family? Obviously many influences are at work. Part of the problem is that many adults do not know how to resolve their differences effectively, and this has consequences for children. Children are highly sensitive to parents' discord, and there is increasing evidence of negative effects of parents' discord on children's development (Grych & Fincham, 1990).

Conflict and disagreement are byproducts of people living together, a normal part of family life. Working out differences can be constructive, but at the same time, conflict poses challenges for interpersonal relations and has the potential for highly negative outcomes (Pruitt & Rubin, 1986). Typically, the expression of anger elicits negative emotions and induces physiological arousal in adults (Levenson & Gottman, 1983) and children (Ballard, Cummings, & Larkin, 1993; El-Sheikh, Cummings, & Goetsch, 1989). Conflict may quickly escalate to violence, grossly distort interpersonal perceptions, and induce a proliferation of disagreements between the people involved (Pruitt & Rubin, 1986).

Conflicts can become uncontrollable and take on a life of their own. Even well-meaning individuals can fall into the social traps posed by interpersonal conflict, with negative implications for the quality and even continuation of relationships (Myers, 1990). Psychological research plays an important role in discovering answers to the complex questions of how best to handle conflict within families. A hopeful development is that an impressive accumulation of knowledge has occurred in recent years on these questions.

While we are concerned with all aspects of conflict within families, in this book we focus on how children fare in interparental conflict. Much that is new has emerged in the past decade concerning children's coping with adult's anger. Exposure to interadult discord has significant impact on children's emotional, behavioral, interpersonal, and even physiological functioning. In addition, indirect effects of marital discord within families may include changes in parenting practices and other types of parent–child interactions. However, it is not that parents have conflicts that is of concern, since disagreement is a normal and even healthy occurrence within marriages. Rather, *how* the parents fight and whether they are able to resolve their differences probably holds the key to understanding the impact of marital discord on children.

The fact that most parents have only the best of intentions for their children and their marriages is hopeful. A lack of knowledge or awareness is an important, if not the primary obstacle, to more effective family functioning.

While advice about how to handle conflicts within families abounds in the popular culture, it often has little foundation and may even be destructive. By contrast, the results of systematic research on marital discord and child development are not widely known or reported. There is a need for useful, helpful information to be made more widely available and accessible. This volume was undertaken, in part, with this concern in mind.

AN OVERVIEW OF THIS BOOK

This book provides an up-to-date review of research on conflict processes within families, with a special concern for the children's perspective. Thus, we consider the effects of interadult conflict on children and the influence of marital discord on children in relation to broader aspects of family functioning. Also, we examine how, when interadult conflicts do arise, they might be better handled from the perspective of the child.

Chapter 1 considers the long-term impact of marital discord on children and their risk for the development of psychopathology. The social problem posed by marital discord for the healthy development of children within families is clearly established by a large body of clinical field studies. Marital discord is positively associated with the development of behavior problems in intact families (Grych & Fincham, 1990). In addition, marital discord may be an important mediator of the development of psychopathology in children of divorced (Amato & Keith, 1991) and depressed (Downey & Coyne, 1990) parents.

Chapter 2 reviews the research on marital interactions in distressed and nondistressed couples. While work on conflict within the marital dyad only infrequently considers children, it constitutes a vital cornerstone of our general knowledge of the principles and processes of conflicts within families. Dysfunctional marriages provide an impetus for destructive conflicts between the parents, resulting in children's exposure to interparental anger and hostility. This chapter considers conflict styles of distressed marriages, the bases for marital distress, long-term consequences of marital anger and apathy, and ways of fighting for the sake of the marriage.

Chapter 3 considers how children react as bystanders to background anger involving the parents. Background anger refers to anger between adults that children observe as by-standers. Here, as elsewhere in this book, the term "marital" is used for reasons of convenience, but we are concerned with children's reactions to conflicts between any adult partners, whether formally married or not. This chapter documents the emotional, behavioral, and even physiological impact of inter-adult and interparental anger expressions on bystanding children.

An exciting new direction, with implications for an un-derstanding of how parents can fight for the sake of the chil-dren, is work on how children react to different forms of conflict expression and resolution. Chapter 4 discusses re-search on the effects of different ways of fighting, and various forms of resolution or nonresolution of anger, on children.

Chapter 5 examines marital conflict in relation to other individual and family influences. Interparental conflict affects children not in isolation but in the context of multiple family systems and processes. In order to fully understand children's development in discordant families, one must consider the broader pattern of influences on children within the family. In this chapter we examine the specific and interactive effects within the family of marital discord, parent–child attachment, parenting practices, and childrens' own characteristics.

Any meaningful message that one can hope to derive from psychological research is inevitably entwined with method. The methodology of research influences the types of questions that can be asked and the sorts of answers that can be found. In Chapter 6 we make a number of suggestions toward advancing the rigor and diversity of research perspectives in the study of families, conflict, and children, with the hope of stimulating exciting new avenues for research.

Finally, in Chapter 7 we draw some practical implications from the research. These are meant as guidelines for parents and practitioners on how to resolve differences for the sake of the children. Research-based parent education and prevention programs constitute one promising vehicle for communicating more effective conflict resolution strategies to parents. We hope our guidelines will provide some bases for the development of such programs.

In sum, this book treats a variety of themes and issues pertinent to families, conflict, and conflict resolution from the perspective of children. This is the first comprehensive review of these various and timely directions of research on family conflict. As such, this volume provides a general introduction to what is emerging as a new and exciting field of study.

Contents

SIX
Methodology and Message
111

SEVEN
Conclusions, Implications, and Guidelines
131

References
151

Index
189

Children and Marital Conflict

CHAPTER I

Marital Conflict and Child Development

At the outset the extent of the social problem posed by marital conflict and discord merits consideration. Some introductory facts: Approximately 40% of all children born in the late 1970s and early 1980s will experience the divorce of their parents and the often significant interparental hostility and discord that can accompany divorce. Many distressed couples who choose to stay together will continue to exhibit marital conflict and turmoil (Emery, 1982). Marriages are most discordant during the child-rearing years (Belsky & Pensky, 1988; Cox, 1985; Glenn, 1990); marital conflict and discord increase during infancy and early childhood (Isabella & Belsky, 1985; Belsky & Rovine, 1990; Belsky, Spanier, & Rovine, 1983), reaching a peak between early childhood and preadolescence (Anderson, Russell, & Schumm, 1983).

The notion that "problem" marriages increase the likelihood of "problem" children is not new. As far back as the 1930s social scientists reported links between marital discord and psychological problems in children (Hubbard & Adams, 1936; Towle, 1931; Wallace, 1935), and support for this association has been consistent over the years (Baruch & Wilcox, 1944; Gassner & Murray, 1969; Jouriles, Bourg, & Farris, 1991; Porter & O'Leary, 1980; Rutter, 1970).

In the past, research often simply established relations between general marital maladjustment and adjustment problems in children. The findings did not necessarily implicate marital conflict per se as a causal agent. Other aspects of dysfunctional marriages could have accounted for adjustment problems in children, for example, couples' unhappiness with each other, their failure to participate in few outside interests together, and absence of intimate communication between them (Jouriles et al., 1991).

Recent work, however, clearly identifies marital conflict as a key mediator in relationships between marital functioning and child outcomes. First, marital conflict is typical of distressed marriages. Interactions between maritally distressed couples are marked by mutual negativity, escalating anger, and physical aggression (Hotaling & Sugarman, 1990; Markman & Kraft, 1989; Margolin, John, & O'Brien, 1989).

Second, marital conflict is a better predictor of a wide range of children's problems than general marital distress (Emery & O'Leary, 1984; Johnson & O'Leary, 1987; Porter & O'Leary, 1980). Relationships between marital hostility and child psychopathology are clear after statistically controlling for general marital distress (Jenkins & Smith, 1991; Jouriles, Murphy, & O'Leary, 1989).

Third, marital conflict is more closely associated with children's problems than other individual aspects of distressed marriages. Some studies indicate that marital conflict predicts child behavior problems, but covert or "encapsulated" distress between spouses is unrelated to child outcomes (Hetherington, Cox, & Cox, 1982). In addition, overt hostility between parents forecasts child behavior problems better than marital apathy and covert tension (Jenkins & Smith, 1991; Rutter et al., 1974). Thus, of all the problems associated with discordant marriages, marital conflict is emerging as a primary predictor of maladjustment in children.

In this chapter we review the evidence for the negative impact of marital conflict on child development, including the magnitude of the association between marital conflict and children's problems and the specific behavior problems in children associated with marital conflict. Finally, we consider evidence that marital conflict mediates the impact on children of various forms of family dysfunction, including parental depression, divorce, and child abuse.

HOW STRONG IS THE ASSOCIATION BETWEEN MARITAL CONFLICT AND CHILDREN'S BEHAVIOR PROBLEMS?

While marital conflict is a predictor of child behavior problems, not all, not even most, children exposed to marital conflict develop psychological problems. Marital conflict is a common occurrence even in harmonious homes. Further, many children do not develop behavior problems even when exposed to very high levels of marital conflict.

Correlations between child problems and fighting between parents are typically moderate in magnitude. Correlations between the two variables usually range between .20 and .45, although some are as high as .63 (Grych & Fincham, 1990). Thus, marital conflict commonly accounts for 4% to 20% of all of the differences in psychological adjustment problems between children.

On the other hand, few family problems are more closely related to children's poor adjustment than marital conflict, even in "happy" marriages. Anger between spouses is even more closely associated with negative child outcomes in distressed families: Approximately 40% to 50% of children exposed to severe marital hostility (i.e., marital violence) exhibit extreme behavior problems (Jouriles et al., 1989; Wolfe, Jaffe, Wilson, & Zak, 1985), a proportion between 533% and 667% times the behavior problem rates in the general population (Wolfe et al., 1985). Notably, marital conflict is a stronger predictor when family stress is high, that is, among families with (1) low socioeconomic backgrounds (Jouriles, Bourg, & Farris, 1991), (2) a child referred for psychological treatment (Emery & O'Leary, 1982; Grych & Fincham, 1990), (3) a parent with psychological problems (Emery, Weintraub, &

Neale, 1982), and/or (4) disturbed parent–child relationships (Tschann, Johnston, Kline, & Wallerstein, 1989).

WHAT KINDS OF PROBLEMS DO CHILDREN EXPERIENCE IN HIGH-CONFLICT HOMES?

Children from high-conflict homes are more vulnerable to developing some forms of psychopathology than others. The following sections consider these associations more precisely.

Behavioral and Emotional Disturbances

Children from high-conflict homes are especially vulnerable to externalizing disorders, including excessive aggression, unacceptable conduct, vandalism, noncompliance, and delinquency. Between 9% and 25% of the differences between children in externalizing problems is accounted for by marital conflict in the home (Grych & Fincham, 1990). Relationships between marital conflict and children's internalizing problems, such as depression, anxiety, and social withdrawal, are less robust. Commonly, about 10% of the variance in children's internalizing problems is explained by marital conflict (Jenkins & Smith, 1991; Shaw & Emery, 1987, 1988). Some studies report associations between marital conflict and children's externalizing problems, but no relationship between conflict and their internalizing problems (Fauber, Forehand, Thomas, & Wierson, 1990), leading to the significant unanswered question of whether the relatively subtle behaviors that reflect internalizing problems are underreported, which would attenuate the findings.

Social and Interpersonal Problems

High levels of marital conflict also increase the risk that children will develop dysfunctional social skills and relationships (Grych & Fincham, 1990). For example, marital conflict is linked to discordant parent–child relationships (Camara & Resnick, 1989; Forehand et al., 1991; Howes & Markman, 1989; Kline, Johnston, & Tschann, 1991). Degree of marital conflict also predicts teacher reports of poor interpersonal skills and social competence in school settings (Emery & O'Leary, 1984; Long, Forehand, Fauber, & Brody, 1987). Thus, relations with peers may be negatively affected.

Impairments in Thought Processes

Marital conflict is linked to diminished academic performance, manifested by poor school grades and teacher's reports of problems in intellectual achievement and abilities (Long et al., 1987; Long, Slater, Forehand, & Fauber, 1988; Wierson, Forehand, & McCombs, 1988). High-conflict family environments may also affect children's interpretation of social situations and interpersonal relations. Although hard facts are not yet available, a rich theoretical foundation supports the notion that children in high-conflict homes are more likely to view themselves and their social worlds in overly negative and hostile ways (e.g., Davies & Cummings, 1993).

WHAT KINDS OF FAMILY PROBLEMS DO CHILDREN EXPERIENCE IN HIGH-CONFLICT HOMES?

Most studies on the effects of marital conflict on children have sampled relatively normal, intact families. Not surprisingly, links between marital conflict and child difficulties appear to be stronger in samples of families with problems, possibly because children must deal with the "double whammy" of multiple family stressors, including marital conflict (Emery & O'Leary, 1982; Hughes, Parkinson, & Vargo, 1989; Sternberg et al., 1993).

Relatedly, marital conflict may figure prominently in the negative impact of various risk environments on children. Typically, children in a family with a specific dysfunction, such as a parent's depression or alcoholism, are thought to be at increased risk of adjustment problems. The marital conflict associated with a specific parental dysfunction may be a significant but little acknowledged factor mediating certain child outcomes.

Parental Depression

Children with depressed parents are likely to develop a wide range of psychological problems (e.g., Downey & Coyne, 1990). One common assumption is that these problems are caused, either exclusively or primarily by the hereditary transmission of faulty biological structures from depressed parent to child. However, heredity is not the only possible cause for the higher-risk status of children with depressed parents. In fact, biologically based explanations cannot fully account for the association between depression in parents and maladjustment in children (Cadoret, O'Gorman, Heywood, & Troughten, 1985; Reiss, Plomin, & Hetherington, 1991). In particular, biological theories cannot explain why children of depressed parents are more vulnerable not only to clinical depression but to a variety of other mental health problems (Downey & Coyne, 1990).

A number of functional characteristics of families with a depressed parent may contribute to the greater likelihood of negative child outcomes, including parental dysphoric moods, reduced parental responsivity, and insecure parent–child attachment (review in Cummings & Davies, in press). Increased marital conflict in particular may be one of the most salient causal mechanisms.

Heightened parental fighting and aggression are common in families with a depressed parent (Biglan et al., 1985; Coyne, Burchill, & Stiles, 1991; Fendrich, Warner, & Weissman, 1990). In about 30% of couples experiencing marital problems, one spouse is clinically depressed (Gotlib, 1992). The marital problems of these couples are likely to be expressed through frequent and explosive bursts of anger

(Cummings & Davies, in press), violence (Merikangas, Prusoff, Kupfer, & Frank, 1985; Webster-Stratton & Hammond, 1988), and mixtures of anger, dysphoria, and withdrawal (Biglan et al., 1985; Hops et al., 1987; Jacobson, Holtzworth-Munroe, & Schmaling, 1989).

Considerable evidence now suggests that marital conflict plays a significant role in the transmission of psychological problems from depressed parent to child (Cummings & Davies, in press). Some studies show that the combination of parental depression and marital discord better predicts child behavior problems than either factor alone (Shaw & Emery, 1987, 1988); others report that marital conflict is a stronger predictor of adjustment problems in children than parental depression (Keller et al., 1986; Rutter & Quinton, 1984) and that marital discord largely accounts for the relationship between parental depression and children's psychological problems (Emery et al., 1982; Miller, Cowan, Cowan, Hetherington, & Clingempeel, 1993). On the basis of a thorough review of the literature on children with depressed parents, Downey and Coyne (1990) concluded that "marital discord is a viable alternative explanation for the general adjustment difficulties of children with a depressed parent" (p. 68).

Other evidence suggests that marital conflict is most important as a predictor of specific forms of childhood disturbances, in particular externalizing problems. Thus, marital conflict mediates the relationship between parental depression and children's conduct problems but has little effect on the development of internalizing problems. Downey and Coyne (1990) speculated that "marital discord directly increases children's risk for externalizing problems, whereas parental depression has its primary impact on children's risk for depression" (p. 66).

Child Abuse

Parental aggression toward children is strongly associated with interspousal aggression (Gelles, 1987; Hughes, 1988; Jouriles, Barling & O'Leary, 1987). Approximately 40% of the children who are victims of parental physical abuse are also witnesses to spousal violence (Straus, Gelles, & Steinmetz, 1980).

Witnessing spousal abuse alone may contribute to children's vulnerability to behavior problems. Children who are *witnesses* of parents abusing one another exhibit problematic behaviors that are similar to those of children who are *victims* of parental violence (Jaffe, Wolfe, Wilson, & Zak, 1986). In addition, some research indicates that children who are *both* witnesses to marital violence and victims of parental abuse exhibit higher levels of parent-reported externalizing problems than do children who are *either* witnesses or victims of parental violence (Sternberg et al., 1993). High levels of marital conflict have been associated with internalizing and externalizing symptomatology for abused children (Trickett & Susman, 1989). Thus, effects attributed solely to child abuse may also reflect the effects of exposure to spousal violence and conflict.

To date, however, the effects of combined child abuse and marital conflict are not well understood. For example, consistent with an additive model of effects (Shaw & Emery, 1988), marital conflict could have a negative impact on children's behavior that is *independent* of the deleterious effects of child abuse (Hughes, Parkinson, & Vargo, 1989). Alternatively, marital conflict combined with parent–child aggression may *multiply* or *potentiate* children's risk for psychopathology (Rutter, 1981, 1990a). That is, the cooccurrence of interparental conflict and child abuse may have far larger effects than the sum of the stressors considered in isolation. On the other hand, being a victim of parental aggression may be so stressful that its adverse impact overrides any deleterious effects of elevated marital conflict (Grych & Fincham, 1990; also see Sternberg et al., 1993).

Marital Disruption

It is increasingly recognized that the way children function after their parents are divorced depends on the quality of the family environment during the period surrounding the marital separation. One of the most important aspects of the family environment for children whose parents are divorcing is the level of parental fighting. In fact, parental fighting is actually a *better forecaster* of children's functioning after the divorce than the changes in the parents' marital status (from intact to separated to divorced) and the children's subsequent separation from a parent. That is, high levels of marital conflict are more closely related to children's behavior problems than family structure per se (Amato & Keith, 1991; Emery, 1982, 1988; Rutter, 1979).

Marital conflict, moreover, is a salient aspect of family life not only during but before the divorce. Children of divorce commonly have long histories of exposure to elevated parental conflict before the divorce occurs (Block, Block, & Morrison, 1981; Block, Block, & Gjerde, 1988). As many as 11 years before parents divorce, children exhibit heightened aggression, impulsivity, hyperactivity, anxiety, and emotional problems (Block, Block, & Gjerde, 1986). Children's high risk for developing behavior problems before the divorce appears to be a result of the greater marital conflict in their families (Block et al., 1986; Emery, 1988).

Is divorce the best solution from the perspective of the children when there are high levels of conflict between parents? The answer to this question, not surprisingly, is complex (Long & Forehand, 1987). Although some parents put their differences aside after divorce, divorce as a means of escape from conflict is not always effective. Parental conflict often increases upon marital dissolution and continues long after divorce (Emery, 1988; Johnston, Gonzalez, & Campbell, 1987; Long & Forehand, 1987). One study reported that 66% of parental interactions after divorce were characterized by anger and conflict (Hetherington, Cox, & Cox, 1976). Children are sensitive barometers of post-divorce conflict between parents. Children subjected to elevated parental fighting after divorce exhibit more behavior problems than children who experience post-divorce reductions in fighting (Long et al., 1988).

Parental fighting predicts children's aggressiveness and conduct problems during the period of marital dissolution (Emery, 1982, 1988). In fact, stronger links between parental fighting and children's internalizing problems are reported for divorced families than for intact families. Interparental conflict during the marital dissolution relates to childhood depression (Johnston et al., 1987), withdrawal (Johnston et al., 1987; Wierson et al., 1988), inhibition (Jacobson, 1978), low self-esteem (Slater & Haber, 1984), and anxiety (Long, Slater, Forehand, & Fauber, 1988; Slater & Haber, 1984; Wierson et al., 1988). Further, marital conflict appears to be more closely related to internalizing than externalizing disorders in divorced families (e.g., Johnston et al., 1987; Shaw & Emery, 1988; Wierson et al., 1988).

Why the stronger link between parental conflict and internalizing problems in divorced families? One possibility is that marital conflict affects children in combination with other stressful circumstances that commonly occur in divorced homes. For example, parental depression and psychological distress are common responses to marital dissolution. Witnessing both marital conflict and parental psychological distress may increase children's tendencies toward withdrawal, anxiety, and dysphoria.

Another possibility is that children of divorce are exposed to particular types of parental fighting that are strongly related to the development of internalizing problems. For example, divorced parents' arguments often center on child-related issues, such as child rearing or custody (Block, Block, & Morrison, 1981; Johnston et al., 1987). Such arguments create in children feelings of shame and self-blame and fears about being drawn into conflicts (Grych & Fincham, 1993); the last reaction has been linked to depression and anxiety in children of divorce (Buchanan, Maccoby, & Dornbusch, 1991). In divorced families the parents may depend on their children for emotional support or pressure their children into alliances against the other parent. These role reversals and alliance-related stresses may induce withdrawal, anxiety, depression, or other internalizing symptomatology in children (Johnston et al., 1987; Wallerstein & Blakeslee, 1989).

CONCLUSIONS AND CRITICAL QUESTIONS

Parental fighting is a consistent harbinger of adjustment problems for children. Children from high-conflict homes are at risk for a wide range of emotional and behavior disturbances, interpersonal problems, and impairments in thought processes. Conflict between parents may also play a critical but largely unrecognized role in accounting for children's psychological vulnerabilities in families with other salient expressions of discord, such as parental depression and divorce. Thus, marital conflict as a core feature of family life has major implications for the socialization of children.

While the research reviewed in this chapter establishes that a high level of marital conflict is statistically associated with negative outcomes in children, many questions remain.

1. Is conflict between spouses always negative? Are there ways of arguing that contribute to the quality of marriage? What are some of the most destructive elements of conflict from a spouse's perspective? What makes ways of arguing between spouses constructive versus destructive?

2. Does marital conflict directly cause children's psychological problems or is it simply related to other factors (e.g., poor parenting practices) that, in turn, have a direct impact on children's functioning?

3. What are the mechanisms associated with fighting that lead to children's disturbances? In other words, why does marital conflict cause psychopathology in children?

4. Are there ways of marital fighting that are linked with optimal functioning in children or that at least reduce or eliminate negative reactions to interparental fighting? Conversely, are there certain forms of conflict that parents should avoid for their children's sake?

5. What other elements of family life mediate or moderate the impact of marital conflict on child development? Which family characteristics "protect" children from the harmful effects of marital conflict? Conversely, which family problems cooccurring with elevated parental fighting may add to the trauma that children experience?

6. Finally, after all the complexities and controversies surrounding research on family conflict are considered, are there any practical messages to be gleaned from this work? What strategies can parents and clinicians use to maximize the quality of family life?

These are just some of the important questions that we tackle in the remainder of the book.

CHAPTER 2

Conflict in
the Marital Dyad

The ability of marital partners to handle their disagreements is at the heart of the long-term viability of a marriage. The quality of the marriage affects the psychological well-being of spouses and the functioning of spouses as parents.

Marital distress "is the most common reason why people seek psychological help" (Bradbury & Fincham, 1990, p. 3). Marital distress predicts parental emotional distress, depression, negativity and conflict, and violence (Beach & Nelson, 1990; Hershorn & Rosenbaum, 1985; Jacobson, Holtsworth-Munroe, & Schmaling, 1989; Levenson & Gottman, 1983; Margolin & Wampold, 1981). These problems in parents challenge and stress the children and increase their risk for psychological maladjustment (Cummings & Davies, in press; Davies & Cummings, 1993), issues we return to in later chapters.

Thus, the quality of the marital relationship affects the quality of family life. Harmony and satisfaction between the adult partners in families is clearly desirable. However, marital discord and dissatisfaction are increasing (Glenn, 1987), with couples divorcing at about a 50% rate (Markman & Kraft, 1989). Clearly more needs to be done to help marriages and families, including effective dissemination of social science knowledge that advances understanding of problems.

Unfortunately, the public is exposed to a great deal of misinformation and noninformation about marital conflict and divorce. Popular opinion and social trends often serve as the basis for marital advice. For example, in the 1970s and 1980s the cultural trend was the rights of the individual over values of commitment, stability, and obligation in social relationships (Bellah et al., 1985). There was much talk of *me* and little talk of *we* in marriage. For some mental health professionals the concern was not "saving the marriage" but rather helping "spouses achieve whatever is best for them as individuals" (Lear, 1991, p. 60). Marital dissolution and divorce were advocated as a solution for marital problems (Medved, 1989; Smolowe, 1991).

Predictably, divorce sometimes had unanticipated negative consequences, particularly in families with children (Whitehead, 1993). Freedom from the marriage contract does not necessarily mean emancipation from the emotional stress and conflict of a distressed relationship. The making and breaking of affectional bonds is not to be taken lightly (Bowlby, 1973, 1980). Children, although not always adversely affected, do not easily adjust to the changing family relationships, conflict, and disruptions surrounding divorce (Amato & Keith, 1991; Hetherington et al., 1992; Wallerstein & Blakeslee, 1989).

The pendulum is swinging back. In the 1990s, maintaining family stability and commitment is again emphasized. Benefits should ensue from this shift back to responsibility toward others—including one's children. However, there are no easy answers. For instance, divorce in physically abusive marriages may protect the victim's physical and psychological well-being—and even preserve the victim's life (Margolin, 1979; Rosenbaum & O'Leary, 1986). But it is not enough that "commitment and stability are suddenly *back in style*" (Lear, 1991, p. 60, emphasis added), there must be an understanding of how to help marriages and families work better.

The effective communication of research findings to the public should be an important goal (Beutler, Williams, & Wakefield, 1993), and some laudable efforts are being made (Baucom, Sayers, & Sher, 1990; Greenberg & Johnson, 1988;

Markman & Kraft, 1989). However, much more needs to be done. Sound information is not widely disseminated or emphasized; witness the psychobabble that dominates many talk shows on television.

In this chapter, and throughout this book, we consider scientifically based information about marital functioning and the effects of marital functioning on children. While the focus of the book as a whole is on the impact of marital discord on children, since marital conflict begins with the parents, an understanding of the origins, causes, and processes of marital conflict from the parents' perspective is important to a complete understanding of conflict processes within families.

This chapter considers conflicts within marital dyads—the pitfalls, problems, and possible solutions—based on scientific studies on these questions. Several themes are considered: the anatomy of a distressed marriage, the causes of marital distress, the consequences of marital anger and apathy, gender differences in conflict styles, and ways to fight for the sake of the marriage.

ANATOMY OF DISTRESSED MARRIAGES

Negativity is the hallmark of a distressed marriage. More negative interactions occur between distressed than nondistressed spouses (Bradbury & Fincham, 1992; Krokoff, Gottman, & Roy, 1988; Levenson & Gottman, 1983; Markman & Kraft, 1989; Smith, Vivian, & O'Leary, 1990).

One thinks of people "getting used to" things that frequently occur. However, spouses do not habituate to anger expressions by their partners in distressed marriages. Instead, hostile reactions are more likely to occur (Jacobson & Margolin, 1979; Margolin & Wampold, 1981; Margolin, John, & O'Brien, 1989). As distress increases, marital partners become *sensitized* to anger and conflict.

The spouses' degrees of freedom in interaction are reduced when they have a history of marital distress. Once a fight starts it is more likely to continue. Reciprocal negativity is characteristic, so each spouse responds with anger to the other's anger (Bradbury & Fincham, 1987; Gottman, 1979; O'Leary & Smith, 1991). Marital conflicts are more prolonged, and there is greater enmeshment in anger and conflict. Fighting in future interactions is more likely.

Escalation and the Kitchen Sink

Conflict escalation is common in distressed marriages (Krokoff, Gottman, & Roy, 1988; Levenson & Gottman, 1985; Margolin, John, & O'Brien, 1989). Spouses do not simply mirror each others' negativity; they raise the level of anger as the fight continues.

Unresolved problems from past conflicts are brought up, a proliferation of issues called "kitchen sinking" (Markman & Kraft, 1989). Added shortcomings, criticisms, and problems are raised as conflicts continue and escalate, fueling feelings of anger and despair and detracting from the possibility of resolution. Old and new issues often remain unresolved.

Consider the following real marital argument, taken from the television documentary *Couples Arguing* (Gantz & Gantz, 1985):

WIFE: (*a little angry*) What is the big deal for you to wait five or ten minutes and let me read a little bit? Why isn't that okay?

HUSBAND: (*a little angry*) I wanted to go to sleep and I couldn't go to sleep because the light was on.

W: What's five minutes?

H: Ann, what do you mean what's five minutes? I told you—

W: (*interrupting, with increasing irritation*) It's preposterous . . . I wanted to read.

H: You are. . . . You can do anything you want to.

W: And you don't even talk to me. You don't give me a chance. You just throw out these ultimatums, and get violent, and get angry, and you just slam doors, and you just say to me, "You don't do what I want and I'm leaving—"

H: (*angrily interrupting*) No, or else I'll sleep out here. So I come out here to sleep and you come out and follow me. And start making it impossible for me to rest—

W: (*interrupting with escalating anger*) I told you a million times that that is really hurtful to me when you do that. And you say, "Okay, I won't do that, I know it's hurtful." You told me before you wouldn't do that and you do it anyway.

H: (*very angry*) You can't decide for me how I'm going to fight with you; what space I'm allowed to have. It's not your decision, it's my decision.

W: (*now very angry as well*) What good does it do to be in a relationship if you can't know my vulnerable points and you can't try to be more careful with them? What good is it to be close to someone if I can't have you being careful with a part of me that hurts more? What good is it then? Why don't you ever respect those parts of me?

H: I don't acknowledge that I never respect any parts of you that are vulnerable, Ann. I feel like I walk around you, and you expect everything.

W: (*submitting while expressing sadness*) I don't think that's true.

This dialogue is typical of "kitchen sinking." A disagreement over late-night reading blossoms into a more intense conflict over more significant marital problems: the husband's lack of sensitivity and the wife's neediness and demandingness. In the end, the underlying anger and sadness remain and the problems, large and small, are unresolved.

Violence

Interspousal violence is linked with certain types of anger expression in marital conflicts (Lloyd, 1990; Maiuro, Cahn, Vitaliano, Wagner, & Zegree, 1988; Markman, Duncan, Storaasli, & Howes, 1987). One study reported that 95% of the women who experience physical abuse also experience psychological abuse, including threats of harm, ridicule, and verbal abuse (Follingstad, Rutledge, Berg, Hause, & Polek, 1990). Escalation during conflict is associated with violence (Jacobson & Margolin, 1979; Hotaling & Sugarman, 1990; Rosenbaum & O'Leary, 1981). Violent couples engage in more heated, prolonged conflicts (Lloyd, 1990), with more verbal abuse, yelling, and threatening gestures (Margolin, John, & Gleberman, 1988; Margolin, John, & O'Brien, 1989).

The potential dangers of highly emotional, angry marital exchanges are not always appreciated, even by therapists. One popular technique for intervening with maritally distressed couples is to encourage the verbal and physical expression of anger. This is intended to be cathartic, reducing anger and frustration (Steinfeld, 1986). However, high levels of anger expression *increase* not decrease, marital violence (Berkowitz, 1983, 1989). A better strategy is to try to stop the escalation of anger and conflict in marital interactions, which reduces the probability of interspousal aggression (Rosenbaum & O'Leary, 1986).

Apathy and Alienation

Spouses may instead react to marital problems with indifference, withdrawal, and disengagement from the relationship (Christensen & Shenk, 1991; Gottman, 1979; Ilfeld, 1980; Margolin & Wampold, 1981; Pearlin & Schooler, 1978; Whiffen & Gotlib, 1989). Withdrawal is a natural and sometimes adaptive response to potentially destructive interactions. It is desirable for couples to withdraw from anger and conflict when marital interactions become heated. But distressed couples become withdrawn and distant even during discussions that would typically be considered benign (Chelune, Waring, Vosk, Sultan, & Ogden, 1984; Christensen & Shenk, 1991).

It is not always the case that both partners are demonstrative or withdrawn. Sometimes one partner becomes overtly angry and the other withdraws. This is called the demand–withdraw pattern. The demonstrative spouse presents grievances and criticisms, and the partner, in turn, becomes passive and defensive (Christensen & Heavey, 1990; Greenberg & Johnson, 1986, 1988; Markman & Kraft, 1989).

CAUSES OF MARITAL DISTRESS

In distressed marriages conflict becomes increasingly predictable, as if it takes on a life if its own. What fuels destructive conflict? What can lead initially well-intentioned spouses into becoming angry cocombatants?

Incompatibility

Incompatibility is one contributor to marital distress (Freed & Foster, 1981; Welch & Price-Bonham, 1983). For example, the demand/withdraw style has been described as a "symptom" of spousal differences in the preference for intimacy versus closeness (Greenberg & Johnson, 1988). Spouses who crave more intimacy may nag and criticize their partners to elicit more involvement. In turn, partners valuing independence respond to such behaviors as a threat to their personal autonomy and withdraw and distance themselves to maintain their independence (Christensen, 1988; Jacobson, 1989).

Incompatibility in the need for intimacy has the potential to exacerbate conflict and minimize positive interaction. Constructive communication between spouses has been found to be negatively related to differences in preferences for intimacy (Christensen & Shenk, 1991). However, spousal differences are only modest predictors of marital problems in themselves (Fincham & Bradbury, 1987; Gottman, 1979); virtually every couple has some differences about money, sex, in-laws and other everyday concerns (Lloyd, 1990; Margolin, 1979).

"How It Should Be" Is Not Always "How It Really Is"

Individuals bring certain beliefs about "normal" spousal relations and roles to their relationships. When these standards are inconsistent with actual marital relations, anger, distress, and negativity in the marriage may result (Bradbury & Fincham, 1989; Eidelson & Epstein, 1982; Markman, Floyd, Stanley, & Jamieson, 1984).

Beliefs create self-fulfilling prophesies. For example, the belief that "men are faithless" fuels a wife's mistrust and negative interpretation of her husband's behavior, increasing her anger and dissatisfaction with the marriage (Baucom & Sayers, 1989).

When one spouse believes that the other's disposition won't change, hostility, defensiveness, and withdrawal ensue. Pessimisism about the marriage and a desire to terminate it may follow (Epstein & Eidelson, 1981; Epstein, Pretzer, & Fleming, 1987). The associated sense of helplessness and lack of incentive to work toward improvement impairs the potential for resolving marital problems. Marital problems then accumulate.

The belief that the partner should be able to read minds and sense needs, even without explicit communication, also predicts negative marital outcomes (Eidelson & Epstein, 1982). For example, a husband may interpret his wife's lack of responsiveness as selfishness when, in fact, he has not adequately articulated his needs (Fincham & Bradbury, 1987; Bradbury & Fincham, 1988). Persistent negative attributions about the wife may follow, along with feelings of disappointment, despair, and being misunderstood in the marriage.

In some relationships any disagreement, no matter how trivial, is interpreted as signaling a lack of love and as a serious threat to the relationship, with the partners experiencing anger and feelings of alienation (Eidelson & Epstein, 1982; Epstein & Eidelson, 1981). Among such couples even minor, infrequent disagreements can have a significant negative impact.

Marital belief systems can be an outcome as well as a cause of marital distress. For example, marital distress may foster distorted beliefs rather than vice versa. Also, distorted belief systems may shape marital conflict indirectly rather than directly. For example, unrealistic expectations may foster negative attributions about the spouse, leading to dysfunctional marital relations (Fincham & Bradbury, 1987).

Communication Breakdown: When the Message Intended to Be Sent Is Not the Message Received

How couples handle differences is also important in marriages (Margolin, 1979; Markman & Kraft, 1989). Dysfunctional communication styles have repeatedly been shown to be associated with marital distress (Bradbury & Fincham, 1992; Margolin & Wampold, 1981; Markman et al., 1987).

Getting a message across is a complex process consisting of a chain of communication events (Bradbury & Fincham, 1990; Noller & Fitzpatrick, 1990), illustrated in Figure 2.1. First, the speaker conceives of a message. Next, the speaker expresses the message, which may or may not reflect the intended communication. The partner then attends to part or all of the message and interprets the meaning of the message; the interpretation may or may not reflect the true intent. The partner then responds, and the communication process returns to the spouse. There is thus ample opportunity for communication errors, which have the potential to maintain or contribute to marital distress.

Problems Sending and Receiving the Message

Communication is more than simply verbal content; it also consists of facial expressions, gestures, and tone of voice. In some studies nonverbal expressions have emerged as better barometers of marital distress than the verbal content of interactions (Gottman, 1979; Gottman, Markman, & Notarius, 1977).

When distressed spouses send a positive message, negativity may leak out in negative tone of voice, gestures, and facial expressions (Noller, 1987). Negative nonverbals can in themselves induce anger in the partner, setting up an ensuing conflict.

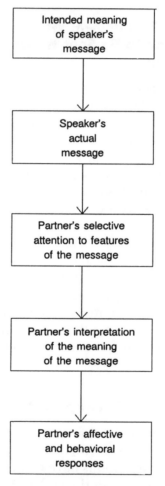

FIGURE 2.1. A model of the marital communication process.

Even if the intended message is sent, the partner may not accurately receive it. Spouses frequently perceive and remember events differently; husbands and wives disagree more than half the time about the occurrence of marital events for a given day (Baucom, Epstein, Sayers, & Sher, 1989; Jacobson & Moore, 1981). This is a particular problem in distressed marriages (Christensen & Nies, 1980; Gottman & Porterfield, 1981; Robinson & Price, 1980). Distressed partners may pay selective attention to negative spousal behaviors, which is called "negative tracking" (Baucom & Sayers, 1989; Fincham & O'Leary, 1983; Jacobson & Margolin, 1979). Even when the message is largely positive or neutral, the negative features of the message become the focus (Notarius, Benson, Sloane, Vanzetti, & Hornyak, 1989).

The impact of communication is determined not by the partner's actual behavior but by spousal perceptions of partner behavior. Spouses who perceive their partner's behavior as positive are likely to respond with positive behaviors. Conversely, when spouses perceive their partner's messages as negative, they react negatively, regardless of whether the partner's actual behaviors were positive, negative, or neutral (Gaelick, Bodenhausen, & Wyer, 1985; Notarius et al., 1989). Negative tracking may be a powerful factor in fostering or maintaining interspousal anger and hostility.

Problems Interpreting the Message

Spouses in distressed marriages interpret their partner's behavior in more hostile ways than do happy couples (Markman et al., 1984; Markman & Kraft, 1989). They tend to accentuate negative partner behaviors and downplay or disregard positive behaviors (Bradbury & Fincham, 1990). Consider the following example:

John, on returning home from work, walks into the living room where his wife Laurie is watching television. Laurie responds with obvious concern in her voice, "Hi, honey,

you're running late. I was getting worried about you."
John, already on edge after a long hard day at work, responds irritably, "Geez, I'm not that late. I've worked this
late before and it didn't seem to matter."

This appears to be a harmless interaction. However, hostile,
angry thoughts could lurk beneath the surface. Laurie might
interpret her husband's irritability as caused by his bad temper
and negative disposition rather than job stress or fatigue. Similarly, John might attribute Laurie's expression of concern to
her (supposed) basic insecurity and fundamental inability to
trust people. By contrast, spouses in happy marriages more
often attribute negative behaviors to situational pressures
(Fitchen, 1984; Holtzworth-Munroe & Jacobson, 1985; Kyle &
Falbo, 1985).

In distressed marriages, spouses are more likely to interpret specific situations as having broad implications and as
indicating chronic problems. Happy couples tend to judge
instances of negative behavior as infrequent, unconnected oc-
currences (Baucom, Sayers, & Duhe, 1989; Newman & Langer, 1988) and as affecting small, specific areas of marital relations (Camper, Jacobson, Holtzworth-Munroe, & Schmaling,
1988; Fincham, 1985; Fincham, Beach, & Nelson, 1987).

Spouses in distressed marriages negatively color even perceptions of positive events (Fincham & O'Leary, 1983). For
example, if John surprises Laurie with a bouquet of flowers,
Laurie might attribute his gift giving to "his tendency to mind-
lessly follow his boss's advice to buy flowers" and disregard the
possibility that "John is a generous person" (Kyle & Falbo,
1985; Holtzworth-Munroe, & Jacobson, 1985). Further, Laurie might see the gift as "a rare event" with "little bearing on
improving any aspect of their relationship." Happy couples
perceive positive partner behaviors as being stable over time
and attribute such actions to the positive personality of the
partner (Bradbury & Fincham, 1990).

Underlying motives and blame are also evaluated differently in distressed and nondistressed marriages. In compa-

rison to nondistressed couples, distressed spouses perceive their partners as more selfish and blameworthy (Baucom et al., 1989; Fincham, Beach, & Baucom, 1987; Madden & Janoff-Bulman, 1981; Margolin & Weiss, 1978). They also tend to focus on the possible negative causes of the spouses' behavior (Bradbury & Fincham, 1990).

Hostile interpretations may result from a long history of problems with a spouse, that is, a spouse's negative thoughts may accurately represent the partner's actions, which may in fact reflect negative, selfish motivations (Baucom, 1987; Bradbury & Fincham, 1989). Conversely, hostile cognitive sets may foster or maintain negative behavior (Bradbury & Fincham, 1988; Newman & Langer, 1988); specific negative attributions (e.g., blame, negative intent) are linked with specific negative behaviors (e.g., criticism, hostility, defensiveness) (Bradbury & Fincham, 1992; Doherty, 1982; Fincham, Beach, & Nelson, 1987; Holtzworth-Monroe & Jacobson, 1985). Under laboratory conditions designed to foster negative interpretations of partner behavior, distressed spouses exhibit greater anger in marital interactions than do happy ones (Fincham & Bradbury, 1988).

Over time, the cycle of negative attributions and negative behavior may take a toll. Hostile interpretations of partner behavior predict subsequent chains of spousal negativity (Bradbury & Fincham, 1992; Halford & Sanders, 1990) and declines in overall marital adjustment one year later (Fincham & Bradbury, 1987).

Behavioral Contingencies

Angry interactions are unpleasant and stressful. Thus, any behaviors that reduce the immediate aversiveness of these interactions are maintained through negative reinforcement. Unfortunately, effective ways to reduce hostility in the short term can foster greater problems in the long run.

One strategy for terminating conflict is to escalate the level of hostility. If, in the face of such negativity, one partner withdraws or submits, not only is the behavior of the aggressor rewarded, but the victim is negatively rewarded with escape from the spouse's anger. Over time this pattern contributes to a maladaptive style of pursuit by one spouse and withdrawal by the other (Markman & Kraft, 1989).

If both partners escalate their hostility, a cycle of negative reciprocity may develop (Gottman & Levenson, 1986; Jacobson & Margolin, 1979; Margolin, John, & Gleberman, 1988; Markman & Floyd, 1980). Again, negative reinforcement occurs when one partner finally submits.

Finally, mutual avoidance of the occurrence of anger and other expressions of negativity can be rewarding in the short term. However, in the long term a maladaptive pattern of noncommunication and withdrawal may develop (Gottman & Krokoff, 1989).

THE LONG-TERM CONSEQUENCES OF MARITAL ANGER AND APATHY

Anger expression, escalation of hostility, or withdrawal from conflict may terminate conflicts or hold other gains in the short term. However, in the long term, these behaviors do not bode well for marriages.

Anger and Apathy

Spousal disengagement and withdrawal are associated with concurrent marital distress (Gottman & Krokoff, 1989; Menaghan, 1982; Pearlin & Schooler, 1978) and marital problems as many as three years later (Gottman & Krokoff, 1989; Levenson & Gottman, 1985). In fact, the negative consequences of these behaviors may become even more evident over time. One study reported that spousal disengagement was unrelated to concurrent relationship distress but that it predicted difficulties 18 and 30 months later, even after statistically controlling for initial relationship problems (Smith et al., 1990).

Anger escalation also has harmful consequences for subsequent marital functioning. Levenson and Gottman (1985) longitudinally followed up on marriages in which the spouses frequently engaged in conflict escalation. Several ways of fighting predicted declines in marital functioning three years later, including the wives' reciprocation of the husbands' negative emotions during arguments, the wives' persistent pursuit of conflicts with their husbands, and efforts by husbands, in turn, to withdraw.

Mechanisms

Why do certain conflict styles lead to negative outcomes for marriages? There are several theoretical explanations.

Failure to Resolve Disputes

Avoidance and withdrawal indicate a lack of commitment to and disengagement from the marriage (Pearlin & Schooler, 1978). Avoidance, by definition, prevents the resolution of problems. Thus, over time unresolved marital problems accumulate and marital distress increases.

Intense anger and escalation can also decrease the likelihood of conflict resolution. The goal of resolving the original problem may get lost or seem trivial in an increasingly negative context of anger and insult exchange (Billings, 1979; Koren, Carlton, & Shaw, 1980). Again, unresolved marital problems are likely to accumulate, increasing the likelihood of continued marital discord (Jacobson & Margolin, 1979).

A Sense of Helplessness

As efforts to resolve marital disagreements are thwarted, a sense of frustration, helplessness, and hopelessness may develop. Spouses increasingly feel that they will never be able to resolve their differences, regardless of what they say or do (Madden & Janoff-Bulman, 1981). Differences that used to be "resolvable" become "irrevocable." A lack of efficacy or confidence that problems can be weathered together may cause spouses to withdraw and disengage, resulting in accumulating feelings of misunderstanding, alienation, and dissatisfaction (Doherty, 1981a, 1981b; Gottman & Krokoff, 1989; Markman, Floyd, Stanley, & Lewis, 1986).

Negative Spousal Thoughts

Negative marital experiences increase negative cognitions. Bradbury and Fincham (1989, 1990) argue that interspousal conflict patterns do not directly determine overall marital functioning. Rather, negative ways of interpreting spousal events mediate the relation between conflict patterns and marital distress. In other words, negative marital interactions lead to hostile perceptions, which in turn lead to long-term discontent with marriage.

GENDER DIFFERENCES IN CONFLICT STYLES

Although it is controversial, evidence suggests that men and women differ in the ways they engage in marital conflict, particularly when marital ties are tenuous. Therapists report that wives commonly complain that their husbands have difficulty dealing with conflict and intimacy, while husbands complain that their wives are too expressive and emotional (Markman & Kraft, 1989). Further, wives may pressure their husbands with complaints and criticisms, and their husbands in turn withdraw and try to avoid marital disagreements (Christensen & Shenk, 1991; Floyd & Markman, 1983; Levenson & Gottman, 1985; Notarius et al., 1989).

   As an illustration, consider the interactions of another couple from the television documentary *Couples Arguing*

(Gantz & Gantz, 1985). In the interview the husband and wife discuss their general styles of handling disagreements.

WIFE: We kept having, you know, these repeated arguments, and it's like the time between them, you know, became less, and I can't speak for Bill, okay, but I didn't have much time to heal.

HUSBAND: And I had to get up very early the next morning; five o'clock, to go to work. And, eh, I asked her could we just end it tomorrow, everything might be worked out. No, she wanted to pursue it.

W: It hadn't even started out that bad. You know, it was kind of mediocre. But he went and slept in one of the other rooms.

H: She wouldn't let me go to bed early. She was constantly coming into my room, the bedroom I was sleeping in, and thinking we could resolve it; could we do this? And I said, "No, I don't feel good about you now. I've asked you to go to sleep, you're not doing that. You're not doing anything I'm asking you to do."

W: He said, "Can't you just go into the other room and sleep, and tomorrow will be okay?" And I said, "You know, I'm standing here and I know with every fiber of my being that that would be the best thing for me to do." I said, "And I can't do it." I said, "And I don't know why." And it was like I had to push it, knowing that it's gonna make things be worse.

H: She says, "Well I can't sleep until we resolve this." And I said, "Well, you don't need to sleep, I'm the one whose going to work tomorrow—"

W: And you know, at one point I got so frustrated that I opened up the window and just went out on the roof. And he just, I mean, you know, threw up his hands and, umm, went out in the backyard.

H: I ran downstairs and stood out in the backyard and said,

"Jump, I'll catch you. Go ahead, go for it." And, eh, actually that kind of defused the situation because it made her laugh.

W: And I wasn't gonna jump off. You know, but I'm starting to realize that he doesn't know that, you know. I mean, and when I make these dramatic plays that I know what I'm doing and I know what's going on, but nobody else does. I mean as far as they're concerned, you know, I'm desperate and I'm real about it. So, that's what happened with that one, but I don't remember what it was about. When I get to that point, I'm not doing it over an issue, it's just, it's the inability to be heard.

H: She would want every problem to be immediately resolved. Minor or major. And I take the view that some things can go away. You don't have to throw everything aside and resolve everything. And, eh, of course, the problem lies in that what I would consider minor, she would consider major.

In her concluding comments, the wife summarizes: "If he has a bad day, or something's going on and he doesn't want to interact, he withdraws. And I have a hard time with that because I think I've done something. And so I try to find out what's going on. And you know, he doesn't want to communicate, he wants to be alone. And so I keep pushing and he withdraws more, and it just escalates."

Why would men withdraw and women pursue during conflict? (Of course, there are cases of women who withdraw and men who pursue.) One possibility is that men and women are biologically built to handle conflicts differently. Specifically, men may be more physiologically reactive to conflict. Men not only become more physiologically aroused during marital fights (Notarius & Johnson, 1982), they also take longer to recover from the dysregulating effects of arousal (Markman & Kraft, 1989).

Men and women may also have different priorities in

marriage. A case has been made for the notion that women are socialized to value intimacy while men are socialized to value independence (Chodorow, 1978). Face-to-face communication about feelings is a form of intimacy. However, because men value independence, they may feel engulfed. In an attempt to re-establish autonomy, men may withdraw from intimate, emotionally charged interactions. In response, women increase attempts to get their husbands to communicate in order to foster greater intimacy. A pattern may develop in which the wife increasingly pressures the husband to communicate and express emotions while the husband increasingly withdraws.

Combine biological and social influences and the result is devastating. According to Markman & Kraft (1989), as conflict becomes more frequent and intense within a distressed marriage, the husband withdraws to reduce the aversiveness of heightened arousal brought about by his reactive biological system. Withdrawal, however, is a direct threat to the wife's valuation of intimacy. Thus, the wife attempts to reestablish intimacy by pressuring the husband through criticism and blame. As a threat to the husband's autonomy and physiological homeostasis, the husband responds through increasing withdrawal. A demand–withdrawal conflict style thus develops within the marriage.

WAYS TO FIGHT FOR THE SAKE
OF THE MARRIAGE

Are there "good" ways to fight? Conflict and anger are in fact inevitable in most marriages (Markman et al., 1984), but conflict can be constructive and valuable, even necessary, in working out marital differences. It is not whether anger occurs that is significant but rather how anger is expressed and dealt with (Madden & Janoff-Bulman, 1981). Finding healthy ways of engaging in conflict and expressing anger is a more realistic and appropriate goal than eliminating conflict from marriages

(Lear, 1991; Rosen, Moschetta, & Moschetta, 1991; Smolowe, 1991).

Toward Negotiation and Compromise

Couples appear to face a no-win dilemma. In the short term, conflict causes tension and stress. However, ignoring and avoiding conflict only temporarily minimizes stress, resulting in greater emotional pain and problems in the long term.

There are reasons for optimism, however. Marriages are strengthened by moderate levels of conflict if the explicit purpose is resolving problems. Spouses who deal with conflict through negotation and compromise are more satisfied with their marriages than other couples (Christensen & Shenk, 1991; Pearlin & Schooler, 1978; Whiffen & Gotlib, 1989).

Such beneficial effects develop slowly but consistently over the course of the marriage. One study reported that negotiation, while not reducing immediate marital distress, was associated with a substantial reduction in marital problems four years later (Menaghan, 1982). Another reported that conflict engagement, while linked with concurrent marital problems, predicted improvement in marital relations three years later (Gottman & Krokoff, 1989). While results may not be immediate, efforts to address differences may strengthen the marriage in the long run.

Toward Successful Resolution

Some couples are successful in resolving problems, whereas for others the hope of achieving mutually satisfying compromises is dismal. What determines whether a couple is successful in resolving their differences?

Establishing a Mutual Awareness

Both spouses need to be aware of the underlying problems. Thus, discussion must occur. However, it is critical that both spouses remain open-minded, empathetic, and flexible. If spouses become defensive or egocentric, their interactions become increasingly angry and aroused (Markman & Kraft, 1989). Further, discussion should not entirely focus on the differences, which may exaggerate the problems. It is important to articulate the marital issue in an open-minded, understandable manner, without too much focus on the negative (Newman & Langer, 1988).

Communication Skills

Some couples do not know the specific skills necessary to communicate in a positive, constructive way. Couples communication has become an important area of study in marital research (Jacobson & Margolin, 1979).

One effective strategy is taking taking turns verbally summarizing the meaning of the partner's messages. This fosters negotiation and compromise by clarifying issues, thus preventing misunderstandings (Markman & Floyd, 1980).

People want to have a sense that they are being understood. This provides a sense of validation and consequently increases the willingness to work toward a constructive resolution of differences (Markman, Floyd, Stanley, & Storaasli, 1988). However, simply listening does not necessarily communicate that one is, in fact, listening. Eye contact, head nodding, a positive tone of voice in responding, and other expressions that clearly show interest can effectively emphasize that one is listening, thus validating the partner's communication (Markman et al., 1984).

Further, the way in which complaints are expressed is important. Sending negative messages (e.g., "You are lazy") during supposedly constructive discussion fosters anger and defensiveness in the partner. Spouses should limit themselves to specific issues and avoid imparting blame (e.g., "I feel like a maid when you come home and leave your shoes in the middle of the living room floor; I'd like it if you could put them in the closet when you are not using them") (Jacobson & Margolin, 1979; Markman & Floyd, 1980).

Giving the Benefit of the Doubt

A persistent tendency to interpret the partner's behaviors negatively is a barrier to any hope for the constructive resolution of differences (Bradbury & Fincham, 1990; Margolin & Weiss, 1978; Newman & Langer, 1988). For example, if a wife perceives her husband's attempts at communication to be motivated by selfish, negative intentions, she will predictably respond with anger, blame, and other negative reactions, regardless of what he says. Giving a spouse the benefit of the doubt provides a foundation for negotiation, even in quite angry fights (Gelman, 1989). Thus, a wife who interprets her husband's yelling as well-meaning and unintentionally negative-sounding, perhaps influenced by job stress, will be more willing to respond constructively to the content of his communications. Discounting the negative partner behaviors and highlighting the positive partner behaviors promote progress toward mutually satisfying solutions to marital problems (e.g., Bradbury & Fincham, 1987, 1990; Margolin & Weiss, 1978; Markman et al., 1986).

Positive perception of the spouse's communications has been linked in research with positive, constructive problem solving during marital disagreements (e.g., Bradbury & Fincham, 1992; Halford & Sanders, 1990). Communication skills training is more successful when programs to change negative styles of interpreting marital events are included (Margolin & Weiss, 1978). On the other hand, efforts at restructuring a spouse's perceptions of the other are not effective in improving marital relations (Baucom, Sayers, & Sher, 1990). Further, benign interpretations are maladaptive if spouses are then motivated to stay with violent partners, putting them at risk for physical and psychological harm (Herbert, Silver, & Ellard, 1991; Holtzworth-Munroe, 1988).

Confidence in the Ability to Work Out Problems

A sense of efficacy about being able to solve marital problems may also foster effective problem solving (Madden & Janoff-Bulman, 1981; Gottman & Krokoff, 1989). Such beliefs can increase the motivation, energy, and persistence necessary to solve marital problems (Doherty, 1981a, 1981b).

Controlling Arousal Levels

Since conflict is a negative, arousing event (Levenson & Gottman, 1983), responses may be guided by anger and "automatic" negative response sets rather than by rational, conscious thought processes (Vasta, 1982). High levels of physiological and affective arousal interfere with rational problem solving (Bradbury & Fincham, 1987).

Several rules and strategies have been developed to help spouses control arousal and thus avoid escalating anger and hostility (Margolin, 1979; Markman & Kraft, 1989; Rosenbaum & O'Leary, 1981), among them time out, stop action, rational self-talk, relaxation techniques, and identifying cues of negative arousal. These strategies, by reducing the occurrence of high levels of anger and arousal, facilitate rational attempts at reaching a constructive resolution to disagreements (Billings, 1979).

SUMMARY AND CONCLUSION

Conflict within a marriage in itself does not indicate marital distress; conflict occurs even in the happiest of marriages. How couples fight and the sources and contexts of the fighting are more significant indicators of marital distress. Avoidance, conflict escalation, and violence are associated with problematic marriages. Unrealistic beliefs about marriage, difficulty in expressing feelings and problems, negative interpretations of the causes and meaning of marital communications and events, and behavioral contingencies also contribute to likelihood of destructive rather than constructive marital conflict. By contrast, couples benefit from constructive conflict processes and strategies that move toward negotiation and the resolution of marital problems.

Children's Reactions to Marital Conflict

When the family consists of only the spouses, dyadic interactions fully describe conflict processes within the family. However, families often include children. Children may be bystanders to the parents' conflicts, or they become participants in the parents' fights as mediators or even as cocombatants. Conflict episodes that initially involve just the parents may quickly become much more complex, involving triadic, quadratic, or even more complex interactions.

Even very young children may be drawn into the parents' fights. In following example, a 20-month-old child is exposed to anger expressed by the mother and father. The mother is the reporter.

> I was very upset about, well, I still had the flu virus and I wasn't feeling very well. And the house was a shambles, where the children had been running and pulling out toys, and the dishes had not been done, and there were clothes on the floor. (They played mommies.) So the house was in bad shape. So I put Clara to bed and I made Tommy go to his room to rest. And then I ran down to the kitchen to put away some of the things that were out of the refrigerator in there, and things that would spoil. And Dick was in the kitchen and I yelled at him, "I don't care if this house stays a mess forever, I am not picking up another damn thing." And I screamed to the top of my lungs, I was mad and I was

furious. . . . And in a squeaky voice . . . I heard Clara say, "Mommy, shut up." She said this about three times. The whole incident didn't last longer than 15 seconds. (Cummings, Zahn-Waxler, & Radke-Yarrow, 1981, p. 1276)

While only a subset of affective communications within the family, interparental anger and conflict expressions are disproportionately powerful events. They may significantly influence children's perceptions of the emotional environment of the home, have an impact on their own capacity for regulating their emotions and behavior, and teach important lessons concerning either adaptive or maladaptive ways of handling conflict.

Another example, also based on the mother's report, illustrates how emotionally arousing and involving the parents' fights can be for children. In this example the child is 6 years old.

My husband John got home late, and I was afraid we were going to miss our plane. I had the children ready and the luggage ready, and I was walking around the house very tense and annoyed. I was muttering to myself and to everybody who'd listen about, well, that we weren't going to make it to the plane and this was terrible. Carl said to me, "You're upset, hah?" and I said, "Yes, I'm very upset at Dad. I don't like being this late." And he said, "Well, I'll go outside and look for Dad." And when John came home Carl said, "Mom's pretty upset, Dad, you shouldn't have been late." And while he was saying this he was sort of jumping up and down and looking a little bit anxious. And then we got into the car and I said to John, "I can't stand this being late; it gives me an ulcer; it's driving me crazy, we'll never make it." He didn't answer or anything and that was the end of the episode. (Cummings, Zahn-Waxler, & Radke-Yarrow, 1984, p. 65)

Clearly, any accounting of conflict processes within families with children must consider the behavior of the children when the parents fight. The children's emotions and behaviors are an important part of what transpires in these contexts.

Relatedly, one must also consider the problems that marital discord creates for children. As we saw in Chapter 1, considerable evidence links marital discord with psychopathology in children (Grych & Fincham, 1990). Children's exposure to marital discord and the response patterns associated with exposure may significantly contribute to the processes through which conflict in the home affects children.

Until recently, the direct impact on children of exposure to and involvement in interparental conflicts received little attention. The focus instead was on the *indirect effects* of parents' fights on children, that is, the sequelae of marital dysfunction that affect children by negatively affecting the ways families function. For example, the stress of interparental conflict can cause parents to become more inconsistent and ineffective in their parenting behaviors, thereby increasing the rate of child misbehaviors (Fauber & Long, 1991). As another example, marital discord may reduce the responsivity of parents to children's emotional needs and signals, thus diminishing the quality of the emotional relationships or attachments between parents and children (Egeland & Farber, 1984; Stevenson-Hinde, 1990) and increasing the rate of various types of childhood problems (Bretherton, 1985). Poor marital functioning may also reduce the quality of sibling relationships resulting in more sibling rivalry and conflict (Brody, Stoneman, McCoy, & Forehand, 1992).

The indirect effects of interparental discord on other relationships within the family (see Chapter 5 for more on this topic), are not the only mechanism of negative influence on children. Repeated exposure to interparental conflict can in itself affect children's functioning. The results are the *direct effects* of marital discord. Clinical field studies and analogue research have consistently shown that interadult conflict is a stressor for children. Exposure to interparental anger may induce emotional distress in children, enmesh them in their parents' problems, or elicit angry or aggressive displays, con-

tributing over time to the development of dysfunctional behavior patterns in children (Cummings & Cummings, 1988).

The importance of children's experiences with adults'
conflicts in the home is still not widely recognized (Emery,
Fincham, & Cummings, 1992). Nonetheless, this chapter focuses on evidence for the direct effects of interadult anger on
children's functioning and development, with particular attention to the potential impact of simple exposure to interparental anger on children. Specifically, we review evidence that
anger between parents is stressful and emotionally arousing
for bystanding children and that it induces in children negative interpersonal behavior, including aggression and involvement in the parents' problems. Further, we consider the possible long-term effects of repeated exposure to parents' fights,
age and sex differences in responding, and the implications of
children's sensitivity and reactivity to adults' anger expressions
for children's development within families.

CHILDREN'S RESPONSES TO MARITAL ANGER: DISTRESS AND EMOTIONAL AROUSAL

Children's emotional sensitivity to background anger, defined
as angry interactions between adults that children observe as
bystanders, is well-documented. Marital discord is one important category of background anger that occurs in homes.

Behavioral Responses

Children frequently, perhaps typically, react with behavioral
signs of distress when exposed to background anger. Research
indicates that the following overt motor responses may occur:
crying, freezing (motionless tension for an extended period),
facial distress, distressed body movements (e.g., covering of
the ears), requests to leave, and verbalizations of discomfort,
anxiety, or concern (Cummings, 1987; Cummings, Iannotti, &

Zahn-Waxler, 1985a). Distress reactions have been reported in observational studies of children's reactions to background anger across a wide age range, from early infancy (Shred, McDonnell, Church, & Rowan, 1991) to late adolescence (Cummings, Ballard, & El-Sheikh, 1991). Among infants and preschoolers positive emotional responses have sometimes been observed as well, but positive responses probably indicate a general arousal of emotions and nervous anxiety rather than happiness (Cummings, 1987).

Children's behavioral responses to background anger are significantly different from their responses to other background emotional interactions between adults (e.g., affection, positive emotion), indicating that children discriminate anger as stimulus. Observations support the notion that background anger induces distress and emotional arousal in children. However, the observation of children's behavior cannot tell us with certainty what children are actually feeling. In other words, covert processes, such as anxiety, cannot be inferred with complete confidence from overt behavior. Thus, a child's freezing when faced with background anger might indicate uncertainty but not necessarily fear or distress. As another example, children may ask to leave a laboratory room simply because they are bored, not because they are afraid.

To convincingly demonstrate that distress is induced in children by exposure to background anger, modes of responding in addition to overt motor behavior need to be assessed (Cone, 1979; Lang, 1968). If a variety of modes of responding to background anger support the same interpretation, then confidence concerning the effects of background anger on children is increased.

Self-Report

Studies of a variety of types of responses support the proposition that background anger induces distress in children and also arouses other negative emotions and behaviors. Some studies have examined children's self-report, that is, asked children how they felt during exposure to interadult conflict. Children often report sadness and anger in response to background anger; younger children in particular sometimes describe fear as a reaction (Cummings, 1987; Cummings, Vogel, Cummings, & El-Shekih, 1989; Cummings, Ballard, & El-Sheikh, 1991). Further, children's emotional reactions are peculiar to anger as a stimulus, that is, their responses indicate that they very clearly discriminate anger from other emotional reactions between adults. Some of the studies that support this point are listed in Table 3.1. More recent work reports that children also describe feelings of guilt, shame, or worry in some contexts, particularly when parental conflicts concern the behavior of the children (Covell & Abramovitch, 1987; Grych & Fincham, 1993). Negative emotional response to background anger has been found in children from 4 to 19 years of age (Cummings, Ballard, El-Sheikh, & Lake, 1991), but of course limited language skills severely limit the feasibility of self-report procedures for children under 4 years of age.

Somatic Responses

A third type of data—somatic responding—is also important in establishing the hypothetical construct of anxiety as a response to parental conflict (Kozak & Miller, 1982). Somatic reactions are significant for interpretations of how exposure to adults' anger affects children, since induced emotional and physiological arousal is a prime candidate as a mediating process between exposure to anger and effects on children's social and emotional functioning (Cummings & Zahn-Waxler, 1992; Emery, 1982). A persuasive case for an "arousal" mechanism as a mediator between exposure to anger and, say, children's aggressiveness (Zillmann, 1983) cannot be made without evidence that children's heart rate, blood pressure, skin conductance, and other physiological reactions are elevated or at least in some way affected by exposure to adults' angry behavior.

TABLE 3.1. Studies of Links between Interadult Anger and Children's
Emotional Arousal

Study	Sample	Comparison	Response
Studies of behavioral emotional responding			
Cummings, Zahn-Waxler, and Radke-Yarrow (1981)	24 children between 10 and 20 months of age; behavior in the home reported over a period of 9 months	Naturally occurring anger > naturally occurring affection	Distress, no attention and response
Cummings, Iannotti, and Zahn-Waxler (1985)	90 2-year-old children	Adults' anger > adults' positive emotions	Distress
Cummings (1987)	85 5-year-old children	Adults' anger > adults' positive emotions	Negative emotions, positive emotions preoccupation
El-Sheikh, Cummings, and Goetsch (1989)	34 4- to 5-year-old children	Adults' anger > adults' positive emotions	Freezing, facial distress, postural distress, verbal concern, anger, smiling, preoccupation
Klaczynski and Cummings (1989)	40 first- to third-grade boys	Adults' anger > adults' positive emotions	Facial distress, postural distress, freezing
Studies of self-reported emotions			
Cummings, Vogel, Cummings, and El-Sheikh (1989)	121 4- to 9-year-old children	Hostile, verbal, and nonverbal anger all > friendly interactions	Negative emotional responses (anger, fear, sadness)
Ballard and Cummings (1990)	35 6- to 10-year-old children	Verbal, indirect nonverbal, destructive, and aggressive anger all > friendly interactions	Anger, distress
Cummings, Ballard, El-Sheikh, and Lake (1991)	98 5- and 19-year-olds	Unresolved anger > partially resolved anger > friendly interactions	Anger, sadness, fear
Cummings, Ballard, and El-Sheikh (1992)	60 9- and 19-year-olds	Hostile, verbal, and nonverbal anger all > friendly interactions	Negative emotional responses (anger, fear, sadness)

Note: From Cummings and Zahn-Waxler (1992). Copyright 1992 by Springer-Verlag.
Adapted by permission.

Several studies indicate that significant changes in children's physiological response systems occur during exposure to background anger, including changes in heart rate (El-Sheikh, Cummings, & Goetsch, 1989; El-Sheikh & Cummings, 1992), systolic blood pressure (El-Sheikh et al., 1989; Ballard, Cummings, & Larkin, 1993), and skin conductance (El-Sheikh & Cummings, 1992). Further, these studies show that somatic reactions to anger are significantly different from reactions to baseline or control conditions; again, it is important to establish that a reaction is peculiar to anger as a stimulus rather than to some other cause. Finally, correlational data suggest links between marital negativity and children's elevated vagal tone in response to stress (Gottman & Katz, 1989).

A limitation on somatic studies is that they are often analogue studies with adult strangers as actors. Gains in scientific rigor are thus offset by questions about generalizability. However, studies of children's reactions to angry parents in the home indicate a generally similar picture of responding (Cummings et al., 1981; Cummings et al., 1984). Further, some analogue studies include parents as participants (J. S. Cummings, Pellegrini, Notarius, & Cummings, 1989a), and others present the parents as the protagonists in hypothetical conflicts (Grych & Fincham, 1993; O'Brien, Margolin, John, & Krueger, 1991). Nonetheless, a fair conclusion is that both interadult anger involving strangers and analogue anger that includes the parents elicit less strong emotional reactions in children than interparental anger in the home (Giacoletti, 1990).

In sum, background anger induces distress and anxiety in children, and this sensitivity to adults' angry behavior begins as early as the first year of life and continues at least through adolescence. Children's behavioral reactions and their self-report support this point. Further, studies of children's physiological responses indicate that interadult anger induces somatic as well as behavioral, cognitive, and emotional arousal in children.

CHILDREN'S RESPONSES TO MARITAL ANGER: INTERPERSONAL FUNCTIONING

An event can induce immediate distress and emotional arousal but not have negative implications for children's long-term development. For example, a child may become upset and aroused by the cries of an infant sibling but learn prosocial lessons from the experience. Thus, a child's disturbance by interadult anger may not mean that long-term negative effects accrue.

A key issue, therefore, is to determine whether interadult anger does result in problematic interpersonal behaviors. Field studies report that children from homes with marital discord are more aggressive (Emery, 1982; Porter & O'Leary, 1980) and enmeshed in familial problems (Block, Block, & Gjerde, 1986; Wallerstein & Blakeslee, 1989), but possibly other variables account for these outcomes. For example, family adversity (e.g., low socioeconomic status, poor social support) could cause both marital conflict and children's behavior problems. The case for marital conflict as a causative agent is strengthened by demonstrations of relations between interadult anger and negative child outcomes under controlled laboratory conditions.

Increased Anger and Aggression

The fact that interadult anger is highly arousing for bystanding children provides a basis for expecting heightened aggression in children. Arousal may translate into increased aggressiveness by means of excitatory processes that continue after exposure to events (Zillmann, 1971, 1982). Direct provocation instigates the transfer of arousal into motivated affective behavior, such as aggression. Contexts that stimulate angry cognitions or affect also increase the incidence of aggression (Berkowitz, 1989). Background anger is both arousing for children and creates an emotional climate for negative and aggressive behavior.

The effects of residual arousal on postexposure actions are not always short-lived (Cummings & Zahn-Waxler, 1992). Repeated exposure to arousal-inducing stimuli prolongs or increases the intensity of response to that stimulus: sensitization occurs (Zillmann, 1983). According to this formulation, a history of exposure to background anger increases children's arousability and thus their proneness to aggression. Rather than desensitizing children to conflict, repeated exposure to interparental conflict has been linked with children's increased emotional and behavioral reactivity (Cummings et al., 1981; J. S. Cummings et al., 1989a).

Exposure to interadult anger might also increase children's aggression because of modeling. Children seldom precisely imitate angry adults (Cummings et al., 1981; Cummings et al., 1985). However, aggressive models weaken children's inhibitions of previously learned negative behaviors (Bandura, 1977). Arousal contributes to modeling: "The disinhibitory power of modeling is enhanced when observers are angered or otherwise emotionally aroused" (Bandura, 1986, p. 291).

Consistent with theory, a series of laboratory studies shows that children's aggression increases following exposure to background anger. One study examined the responses of 2-year-old friends (Cummings et al., 1985). The children played freely while two female actors came and went. First the actors were friendly. Later they returned and became angry at each other. Finally they came back and resolved their dispute. Interchild aggression increased following the 2-year-olds' exposure to the fight and declined again after the resolution. A control group of children exposed to a series of emotionally neutral interactions showed no change in aggression over time.

An example from this study is illustrative. A 20-month-old boy and a 24-month-old girl played together without conflict until the actors became angry. After the actors left, several vividly aggressive exchanges occurred.

> Billy approaches Susan, who is riding a rocking horse. He pulls her backward off the horse. As she gets up he pushes

her and then throws her to the ground. He repeatedly
pushes her backside and then her face to the floor, despite
her crying and screaming. The mothers then intervene.
Minutes later a similar sequence ensues and continues until
the mothers again intervene. (Cummings, Iannotti, &
Zahn-Waxler, 1985b)

These children were seen again in a follow-up study three
years later (Cummings, 1987). As before, interchild aggression
increased following exposure to interadult anger. Aggression
did not increase in the control group exposed to emotionally
neutral interactions. Further analyses indicated that the most
emotionally aroused children were the most prone to increased aggressiveness.

Other studies have replicated these relations. Klaczynski
and Cummings (1989) found that among first- to third-grad-
ers high arousal in response to background anger predicted
increased aggressive impulses towards peers. Another study
reported that physically abused boys became more angry and
aggressive following exposure to background anger (Cummings, Hennessy, Rabideau, and Cicchetti, in press), even
without a peer present. Aggression was directed toward toys,
shown by hostile outbursts, or even aimed at the adult actress.
This study is important because it demonstrated that exposure
to background anger may have pervasive effects on children's
aggressiveness.

Anger and aggression are closely related; anger lowers the
individual's threshold for becoming aggressive (Berkowitz,
1989). Exposure to background anger has repeatedly been
shown to increase anger in children (see Table 3.1), which
increases the likelihood of interpersonal aggression.

In sum, studies demonstrate a causal link between interadult anger and children's anger and aggression. The research supports the notion that exposure to marital discord
can instigate hostility in children, regardless of parenting practices or any other aspects of family functioning.

Increased Involvement in Parental Disputes

The altruism of young children is often underestimated (Radke-Yarrow, Zahn-Waxler, & Chapman, 1983). Even 1- to 2-year-olds may respond to a family member's distress (Zahn-Waxler, Radke-Yarrow, & King, 1979) and comfort, intervene between, and distract parents who are fighting, or in other ways become involved in parental disputes (Cummings et al., 1981).

However, marital conflict is threatening for children, and under "normal" circumstances children have good reasons not to get involved in interparental conflicts. Children risk becoming targets of the parents' hostility themselves. Furthermore, children have very little control over what happens, and thus their actions are likely to be futile. While children may want to help the parents (Covell & Miles, 1992; Grych & Fincham, 1993), their impulses are relatively infrequently translated into action (J. S. Cummings et al., 1989a). Thus, children do not have the motivation or incentive necessary to become directly involved in the parents' disputes—unless the parents are chronically unable to resolve or otherwise handle their disputes themselves.

Children from discordant families have considerably more incentive for taking action than children from harmonious homes (Emery, 1989). Interparental conflicts are more likely to continue for long periods, become progressively worse, become physically abusive, and include the children as targets of hostility (Jouriles, Murphy, & O'Leary, 1989; Wolfe, 1987). If the children's involvement succeeds in reducing conflict or otherwise mitigating negative outcomes, their unlikely behaviors are negatively reinforced, increasing the probability that the behaviors will recur. As the reinforcing process is repeated again and again, children develop a pattern of involvement in the parents' disputes. Again, children's emotional arousal is a factor: The greater arousal and distress induced in children by conflict in chronically discordant homes motivates interventive behaviors (Emery, 1989).

Research demonstrates that children from discordant homes do become more involved in parental disputes. One self-report study reported that, in comparison to other boys, boys from homes characterized by interparental aggression advocated more verbal and physical intervention in the interparental conflicts (O'Brien, Margolin, John, & Krueger, 1991). Another study found that 1- to 2-year olds exposed to much interparental fighting showed greater comforting or distracting of angry parents in the home (Cummings et al., 1981). Even when the expression of anger by adults is controlled under laboratory circumstances, children from homes high in discord often comfort or defend the mother (J. S. Cummings et al., 1989a). In each of these studies children from discordant homes showed more emotional arousal and upset than other children during background anger involving the parents.

A description of the responses of a 5-year-old girl from a home with reported interparental aggression to a laboratory simulation of anger directed at the mother illustrates children's involvement. The mother has seen the script for the actress's angry display and knows it is not real, but she follows instructions to respond naturally.

> As the actress evidences anger at the mother for her negligence in filling out certain forms, Anne shows distress and sadness while looking down at the floor. Play, which has been active, stops and the girl is obviously preoccupied with the angry scene. She looks to her mother occasionally and smiles but the smiles quickly fade. After the actress leaves, Anne gets up and says to her mother, "Doesn't she know that it takes a while to fill out a form?" The child, still clearly distressed, moves to stand near her mother. After a few seconds she sits on the right side of the mother's sofa chair, putting her arm around the mother. She watches closely while her mom fills out the forms, paying special attention to how she is filling them out. She makes several comments: "Is your name on the forms now?" "Are you putting circles on them?" Anne points to specific areas of the forms as she speaks. Finally, she says, somewhat ner-

vously "Are you done with the forms yet?" (J. S. Cummings, Pelligrini, Notarius, & Cummings, 1989b)

The child in this scene is obviously concerned about the mother's welfare; she comforts the mother and takes responsibility for the mother's problems. A few moments later the actress returns and apologizes to the mother in a quite thorough manner. Anne's responses in this instance are also instructive.

> As the apology begins, Anne gets up from next to her mother and goes to the window. As the apology continues, she goes and sits down by her block towers, which are in close proximity to the actress and on the other side of the room from the mother. She plays actively, which she has not done since before the angry exchange. After the actress leaves, the girl says to her mother, "First she's mad, then she's happy." She enthusiastically says to her mother, "How's my building look?" After her mother compliments the towers she comments, "I'm happy that I came, are you?" The mother responds affirmatively and the girl continues to play happily. (J. S. Cummings, Pelligrini, Notarius, & Cummings, 1989b)

The apology by the actress and the obvious reconciliation between mother and actress greatly reduced the distress caused by background anger involving the mother. This is a typical finding and illustrates the importance of how adults fight and whether conflicts are resolved to children's reactions. We will return to this issue in Chapter 4.

Children helping conflictual parents seems laudable and even desirable on the surface. However, taking too much responsibility for the parents' welfare has been linked to dysfunction, and it is burdensome for children (Block, Block, & Gjerde, 1986; Main, Kaplan, & Cassidy, 1985; Wallerstein & Blakeslee, 1989). Also troublesome is the fact that children's oversolicitousness in response to the parents' distress has repeatedly been associated with divorce, depression, and other family disturbances (Cummings & Davies, in press; Emery,

1988). Clearly, in well-functioning families parents ought to take responsibility for the children in times of distress, not the other way around. Thus, increasing evidence shows that it is a cause for concern when children appear "too good" and take responsibility for the parents' problems.

In summary, exposure to interadult anger can have a negative impact on children's interpersonal functioning. Increased aggressiveness and enmeshment in the parents' disputes may result. However, the fact that these effects *can* occur does not mean that they *do*.

IMMEDIATE AND LONG-TERM EFFECTS

Returning to the question of the effects of exposure to marital discord, children's immediate reactions establish that exposure to interadult anger stresses children, affecting a wide range of behavioral, emotional, and social systems. Some of these reactions appear worrisome or problematic. As we saw in Chapter 1, marital discord has been repeatedly associated with negative outcomes in children in field research. However, there is a gap between finding that certain reactions are induced in children and demonstrating relationships between the immediate reactions and long-term development.

This section considers several themes relating children's immediate reactions to background anger with developmental effects. First, reactions are more significant if they can be shown to be part of larger patterns or styles of responding (Cicchetti, 1984; Sroufe & Rutter, 1984). Research indicates that background anger elicits broad-based responding. Second, the developmental implications of response patterns is increased if the patterns are unchanging over time (Waters, 1978). Several studies demonstrate that emotional responding is relatively stable. Finally, response patterns have significance beyond the immediate observational context if they are systematically related to family history (Bretherton, 1985). Numerous studies show that children's reactions to background anger are predictably related to family histories of conflict.

Children's Styles of Coping with Interadult Anger

Children's individual patterns of responding to background anger indicate the exact ways in which children handle background anger in everyday life. Three basic styles of coping with exposure to background anger have been identified: concerned, angry/ambivalent, and unresponsive. These patterns are based on children's responses across multiple response domains: social and emotional behavior; self-report of thoughts, feelings and impulses; physiological responding; and reactions in independent stress-inducing contexts. The following descriptions are based on several investigations of these patterns (Cummings, 1987; Cummings & El-Sheikh, 1991; El-Sheikh, Cummings, & Goetsch, 1989).

The concerned pattern is the most common and suggests adaptive coping. Concerned children show signs of mild distress during exposure to anger between adult strangers (e.g., freezing, distressed facial expressions, and increased heart rate). They report feelings of sadness for the arguing adults and wish they could help them. Appropriately, however, they do not intervene and also do not increase in aggressiveness toward playmates. When faced with the stress induced by separation from the mother, these children behave adapatively, that is, they effectively use the mother as a secure base. In sum, they are mildly stressed by anger and other stressors but handle it well.

Angry/ambivalent children show more signs of difficulty. First, they exhibit more distress and preoccupation in reaction to background anger than do concerned or unresponsive children. Second, in contrast to other groups, they express multiple emotions, including anger, distress, and smiling or laughter. Positive affect in this context is unlikely to indicate enjoyment. Instead, varied and contrasting emotional expressions probably suggest a general activation of emotion systems and arousal. Third, the self-report of angry/ambivalent children suggests out-of-control feelings, for example, crying, wanting to run from the room, wanting to hit the actors. Fourth, these children increase in aggressiveness toward playmates following exposure to background anger, which is incontrovertibly a sign of maladaptive coping. Fifth, their disposition toward aggression following exposure to background anger is stable, reported at both age 2 and age 5. Sixth, angry/ambivalent children evidence decreased heart rate during exposure to background anger. While seemingly a counterintuitive result, lower or dampened autonomic reaction to threat has been repeatedly linked with externalizing behavioral problems, such as delinquency (Lytton, 1990). Seventh, instead of using the mother as a secure base, they avoid the mother on reunion with her following separation. Considerable research indicates that this response is linked with maladaptive social behavior (Bretherton, 1985). In sum, the pattern is one of externalizing problems in coping with stress.

The least common pattern—and the one providing the fewest clues for interpretation—is the unresponsive style. Unresponsive children do not show behavioral signs of distress, nor does their aggression increase. Some may show little reaction because they are not distressed by background anger. On the other hand, when interviewed, unresponsive children report feeling angry at the angry adults. Also, they show the troublesome response of avoiding the mother after separation. From these scant clues one might posit that these children are distressed but are suppressing or internalizing their reactions. Notably, the sadness suggestive of empathy found among concerned children is entirely absent in unresponsive children.

Background anger thus activates many interrelated response systems. The discovery of the three patterns holds the promise of advancing understanding of individual differences in children's adaptive and maladaptive coping with marital discord. Possibly these patterns will provide a window, at a fine-grained process level, into the etiology and behavioral organizational of different types of problems (e.g., externalizing disorders) resulting from exposure to marital discord. However, the clinical significance of these patterns awaits further research specifically testing for such relations.

Stability in Responding to Background Anger

Findings of stability indicate that reactions have import beyond the immediate, transient situation. For example, stability is one requirement for a demonstration of temperament (Buss & Plomin, 1975). A foundation for deriving attachment patterns from infant's reactions to brief laboratory separations from the mother (Ainsworth, Blehar, Waters, & Wall, 1978) is that responses are stable (Waters, 1978).

Research findings repeatedly demonstrate that reactions to background anger are stable over time. One study reported stable distress reactions to laboratory exposures to background anger spaced one month apart (Cummings et al., 1985). Aggressive behavior in this context was also stable. Emotional reactivity is stable over several months for infants (Cummings et al., 1981) and school-age children (Cummings et al., 1984). Most significantly, emotional reactivity to background anger in the home has been reported as stable over a five-year period of early childhood (Cummings et al., 1984). Boys' aggressive behavior in this context is highly stable over a three-year period (Cummings, Iannotti, & Zahn-Waxler, 1989).

In sum, children's reactions to background anger become organized and stable early in childhood.

Family History: The Sensitization Hypothesis

Another form of evidence that responding to background anger has significant implications are relations between reactions to background anger and family conflict histories. Such relations suggest that responses derive from experience.

A common-sense expectation is that children exposed to a great deal of anger in the home would "get used to it," that is, habituate to it. The findings, however, indicate the opposite.

Every study on this question that we are aware of reports that marital discord predicts children's greater reactivity to exposure to background anger (Ballard, Cummings, & Larkin, 1993; Cummings et al., 1981; Cummings et al., 1984; J. S. Cummings et al., 1989; Cummings, Vogel, Cummings, & El-Sheikh, 1989; O'Brien et al., 1991). Further, some particularly worrisome behaviors are elevated, including distress, anger, aggressiveness, and involvement in interadult disputes.

In some of the studies the exposure to background anger is a laboratory presentation that is the same for all children (for example, J. S. Cummings et al., 1989a). Thus, the reactions of children from angry homes may be attributed to their history, that is, their history has resulted in a *sensitization* to marital conflict.

Examples reflecting our various laboratory and home observations illustrate the differences in reactions. Exposed to frequent marital conflict, 1-year-old Susan appears attuned to the parents' distress during their arguments, wiping away the mothers' tears and hugging the mother. Five-year-old John yells angrily when an actor scolds the mother and blocks the door after she leaves in an effort to prevent her return. After an argument between two adults, Joey and Seth fight continuously and with increasing agitation, with Joey finally biting Seth and Seth hitting Joey with a plastic toy hammer. By contrast, same-aged children from significantly less conflictual, angry homes may not even look up from their play during standardized laboratory conflicts, and show no elevation of anger or aggressiveness at any time.

But what of the notion that people habituate to events they observe repeatedly? We suggest that there are at least two levels of responding to repeatedly presented stimuli, an information-processing level and an emotional-conditioning level. At an information-processing level, habituation occurs with repeated exposure to a stimulus. However, at an emotional-conditioning level, we would suggest that sensitization is the process that best describes the cumulative effects of exposure to an emotionally arousing stimulus.

Consider an everyday example. Your worst enemy makes a critical remark about you. You are not at all surprised and learn nothing new. At an information-processing level the event barely registers. Nonetheless, you feel quite aroused and may respond with anger or hostility. A similar remark from a friend might cause surprise but result in only a mild emotional response and no social retaliation.

Thus, the data and some logic support a model whereby repeated exposure to marital discord sensitizes children to the occurrence of conflict. Bases for a sensitization model can be found in other sources. Discordant marital couples show elevated physiological response even before arguing. Histories of discord increase the negativity and likelihood of escalation in disputes (Levenson & Gottman, 1983; Gottman & Krokoff, 1989). In animal studies, traumatic environmental stimuli produce significant changes in social, emotional, and biochemical functioning; providing another parallel to the research on children (Meyersberg & Post, 1979).

An important qualification is that not all conflict histories may be linked with the worrisome patterns of responding. The evidence is that it is most clearcut for interspousal aggression and certain other dimensions of conflict (see Chapter 4). Thus, not just *any* fighting between the parents may foster sensitization. Relatedly, different effects may result from qualitatively different exposure histories. For example, marital discord shown mostly in the "silent treatment" may have quite different effects from marital discord typified by physical hostility. This question has received little research attention.

Children's sensitization to conflict may also be a function of the history of resolution of conflict. In several recent studies children have been exposed either to a couple that always resolves their arguments in a series of conflict episodes or a couple that always fails to resolve their fights. The hypothesis was that repeated exposure to unresolved conflict sensitizes children in relation to the same level of exposure to resolved conflict. Using the procedure, experimental evidence for sensitization as a function of resolution history has been found, particularly among girls (El-Sheikh & Cummings, in press; El-Sheikh & Cummings, 1993).

Returning to the sensitization hypothesis, one can begin to articulate how this process might increase risk for the development of dysfunctional patterns in children. Chronic exposure to conflict and hostility increases children's experienced distress and arousal. Through sensitization, a consequence over time may be further elevated emotional and behavioral acting out and enmeshment in conflict. With the frequent occurrence of conflict these patterns may become a salient segment of the child's behavior and generalize to the child's general repertoire for reacting to stress. Such negative behaviors by children in turn may set in motion a negative pattern of responding in others that increases the persistence of maladaptive patterns (Dodge & Frame, 1982).

Of course, exposure to conflict is only one of many classes of events within the family that affect development; we explore interrelations with other aspects of family functioning in Chapter 5. Repeated exposure to anger is unlikely in itself to lead to behavior problems. Whether children develop psychopathology is likely to be a function of their constitutional dispositions and the exact nature of their family experiences, including the precise patterns of anger expression within the family.

In sum, there is a variety of bases for expecting that responses to background anger have implications for children's functioning beyond the immediate context of exposure. The study of response patterns is one avenue for advancing models of child development in discordant homes.

AGE AND SEX

Are boys or girls more disturbed by exposure to the parents' fighting? At what age do children first react to fighting between the parents? Is there one age at which children are the most vulnerable to exposure to discord? These are among the most-asked questions about the effects of marital discord on children and therefore merit special attention.

Age

A common perception is that young children are not sensitive to interparental communications or emotions. Parents may fight or argue in front of children without regard to their presence, on the assumption that the children will not notice.

The data strongly contradict this view. While young children may well not understand the content of the parents' arguments, they are sensitive to their emotions. Even at 6 months of age children react discriminatively to interadult anger in relation to other emotions (Shred et al., 1991). Children respond to unresolved anger as a stressor throughout childhood (Cummings, Ballard, El-Sheikh, & Lake, 1991; Cummings, Ballard, & El-Sheikh, 1991); they become visibly upset and report emotional reactions of distress or anger.

Reactions do change with age, especially between infancy and middle childhood. For example, toddlers seldom become directly involved in their parents' disputes (Cummings et al., 1981). By school age the disposition to become involved sharply increases (Cummings et al., 1984; J. S. Cummings et al., 1989a), peaking at middle adolescence, according to one study (Cummings, Ballard, & El-Sheikh, 1991). Fear also changes with age; it is most evident at preschool age or before (Cummings, Vogel, Cummings, & El-Sheikh, 1989). Sensitivity to the resolution of conflict greatly increases at about 6 years of age and remains acute for the rest of childhood (Cummings, Vogel, Cummings, & El-Sheikh, 1989; Cummings, Ballard, El-Sheikh, & Lake, 1991).

The findings are not readily interpretable concerning which age group(s) are most vulnerable (Cummings & Cummings, 1988; Hetherington, 1984; Grych & Fincham, 1990). Conclusions are difficult to make for several reasons. First, some responses increase and others decrease with age, and weighing the significance of the increases and decreases to vulnerability is difficult. For example, as children get older they become more emotionally sensitive and involved in discord among family members, which might be seen as increasing risk for mental health problems. On the other hand, they also develop a larger and more effective repertoire of coping strategies, which may well offset the possibly deleterious effects of increasing sensitivity and enmeshment.

Second, research findings are difficult to interpret because exposure history cannot readily be disentangled as a factor. For example, if older children have more problems it could be due either to a more vulnerable developmental stage or to a longer period of exposure to conflict. Only carefully designed studies of children's development over time can decisively address this issue.

Third, at different ages children may be more vulnerable to different types of mental health problems. How does one judge which kind of mental health problem is more important? Age-related vulnerability may be not general but specific to specific types of psychopathology. Young children are vulnerable to externalizing problems—for example, they may respond to stress with aggression, noncompliance, and temper tantrums (Glasberg & Aboud, 1981, 1982). During middle and late childhood children show a higher frequency of internalizing behavior, such as dysphoria and passivity, and depression becomes more prevalent, particularly between late childhood and early adolescence (Angold & Rutter, 1992; Rutter, 1986). Thus, the key question may not be which age is most vulnerable but rather to ascertain the relative vulnerability to specific problems and outcomes at each age.

In sum, children of all ages react to background anger as a stressor, and it cannot be said with confidence that any one age is most vulnerable.

Sex

For a time boys were thought to be more vulnerable than girls to discord, but the issue is no longer clear. Early work reported stronger associations between family discord and behavior disturbances in boys (Robins, 1966; Rutter, 1970). More recent research suggests that the differences between boys and girls may not be so much in the degree of disturbance as in its manner of expression. Consistent with sex roles, boys show dysfunction by increased aggressiveness, whereas girls more often become withdrawn and anxious (Block, 1983; Block et al., 1981, 1986; Cohn, 1991; Emery, 1982). The "too good" child pattern is also more often found in girls. Higher reports of disturbance in boys could simply reflect the greater salience and disruptiveness of their problems and the greater likelihood that the problems will result in clinic referrals (Whitehead, 1979).

Complicating the picture, sex differences in vulnerability may change with age. For example, in divorced families psychological disturbance is more often reported for boys in early and middle childhood, whereas differences in psychopathology are less clearcut in late childhood and adolescence (Hetherington, Cox, & Cox, 1985; Zaslow, 1989)—and perhaps may be the reverse (Werner, 1989).

In terms of childhood responding during exposure to anger, boys have been found to be more prone to hostile reactions and girls more likely to respond with distress (Cummings et al., 1985; Cummings, Vogel, Cummings, & El-Sheikh, 1989). However, some recent research reports that, beginning around adolescence, girls are made more angry by background anger (Cummings, Ballard, & El-Sheikh, 1991), and boys report more sadness (Cummings, Ballard, El-Sheikh, & Lake, 1991).

Putting these findings in perspective, as for many dimensions of psychological functioning more variability probably occurs within than between the sexes, with considerable overlap. Although gender labels foster categorical thinking about differences, in fact sharp differences are seldom found. In any case, the pattern of findings is far from simple and clearly does not justify any certain conclusions about the relative vulnerability of the sexes to exposure to background anger.

SUMMARY

Children are affected by mere exposure to marital discord. Anger between adults, which we term background anger, is stressful and emotionally arousing for children of all ages, and it also increases their aggressiveness. Repeated exposure sensitizes children, increasing their arousal and aggression when exposed to anger and also their tendency to intervene in parents' fights. Children show individual differences in styles of coping with interadult anger and styles are stable over time. Children's styles or patterns of responding to discord may provide clues to their relative vulnerability to the development of psychopathology. While sex and age differences in how children respond to adults' fights have been identified, the evidence is insufficient to conclude that any particular age, or either sex, is more vulnerable to the development of behavior problems.

CHAPTER 4

Effects of Specific Aspects of Marital Conflict on Children

The focus of Chapter 3 on negative effects of exposure to interadult anger should not obscure the fact that most children adaptively respond to parental anger as well as to many other challenges of family life (Garmezy & Masten, 1991). Marital conflict is a stressor in the short term, but it contributes to the development of psychopathology in only a minority of children. Focusing on negative consequences risks pathologizing an event that is non-pathological in many families. Much depends on how often the parents fight and perhaps even more importantly on the ways in which they fight.

Anger is frequently treated as if it were a single or unitary stimulus. In fact, anger and conflict expressions can vary in a variety of dimensions and domains. General awareness of distinctions between different types of fighting is manifest even in the language of the popular culture. One hears of such diverse styles of expressing disagreement as the "silent treatment," a "heated argument," "having words," being "at each other's throat," "gridlock," "talking it out," "giving the cold shoulder," "beating-up," "knock-down-drag-out-fight," "battering," "attacking each other," and giving "looks that kill."

Clearly, discord is expressed in many ways in marriages

and families. Styles of marital conflict may be as important or more important than the parents' level of marital satisfaction to child outcomes (Grych & Fincham, 1990). Even marriages at roughly the same level of distress may, in fact, vary quite widely in patterns of conflict expression, the meaning of conflict for the marriage and the family, and the result of the conflict process. For example, distressed partners may seldom actually talk about the issues troubling them, but nonetheless their feelings may still surface in the form of looks, gestures, and the things that are left unsaid rather than said. In other cases of marital distress highly verbal, emotionally heated exchanges occur, with fights sometimes escalating to include physical violence. These very different ways of indicating marital distress, while perhaps equivalent in terms of the general level of dissatisfaction that is felt by husband and wife, may well have quite different implications for the development of the children.

If couples fight a lot does that necessarily mean that they are unhappy? Some couples have frequent disagreements and disputes but in general feel comfortable with the process of open disagreement and often end things up on a positive note. Do children respond to the parents fighting a lot, or do they take into account the whole picture, including the result of fights?

Disagreements and conflicts between the parents and others in the family are surely inevitable, a normal and natural part of family life. A recommendation that marital partners never fight or get angry is simply not practical and may not even be good advice. Important family issues need to be addressed, in angry and emotional ways at times. Problems that aren't worked out may continue to undermine family relationships and come out in even more destructive ways later (Gottman & Krokoff, 1989). Advice is needed on specific and precise ways of fighting.

From the perspective of the children it is important to know which types of fights are problematic and which are not. What are the effects of different types and ways of fighting?

Which elements of the conflict process are most destructive from the perspective of the child? Can parents do anything to ameliorate the impact of their fights on children?

Relatedly, are there ways for parents to fight that are constructive and even beneficial from the perspective of the child? Parents' conflicts can teach children valuable lessons about how to handle negative feelings and work towards the resolution of interpersonal differences. Parents are potentially valuable role models. Never allowing the children to observe the parents angry or upset could cause children to develop an unrealistic view of the world and relationships, with little preparation for the conflicts posed by real relationships and few of the requisite coping skills. At the other extreme, children from destructively angry homes may learn negative lessons about anger expression and dispute resolution.

In brief, this chapter is concerned with how different ways of fighting affect children and with the implications for the broader question of how the parents can fight for the sake of the children. This is a relatively new area of inquiry, but it is at the heart of understanding the effects of marital conflict on children. First, we consider how different types of anger expressions and resolutions affect children. It is now clear that it matters not only how often the parents fight and how they fight but also how fights end. Second, evidence of links between specific types of anger expression and specific child development outcomes is examined. This evidence is critical to an advanced understanding of the developmental psychopathology of angry environments, since it begins to specify which ways of fighting are associated with negative outcomes or risk for negative outcomes in children. Finally, we end with a discussion of important themes for future research.

CHILDREN'S REACTIONS TO SPECIFIC ASPECTS OF INTERPARENTAL CONFLICT

Interparental conflict can vary in how often arguments occur, the ways in which disagreements are expressed, and the end-result of conflicts. Children are influenced by each of these aspects of marital conflict.

Frequency

Greater frequency of marital conflict is associated with greater difficulties in children (Rutter, 1971). Links have often been reported between frequency of marital conflict and such negative child outcomes as conduct disorders (Hershorn & Rosenbaum, 1985; Jouriles et al., 1991; Long et al., 1987) and academic and other adjustment problems (Emery & O'Leary, 1982; Wierson et al., 1988).

Typically, findings are based on correlational studies of clinic samples. However, correlational findings are subject to alternative interpretations. A third factor (e.g., low socioeconomic status and its associated stresses) could account for both greater marital conflict and more severe adjustment problems in children. Strengthening the case for frequency as a causal influence, studies employing observationally based methodologies also indicate a negative impact of elevated frequency of conflict. Using a diary method in which mothers kept a tally of family conflicts over a nine-month period, Cummings and colleagues (1981, 1984) reported that more frequent interparental conflicts were linked to greater distress, insecurity, and anger in children. Repeated exposure to interadult anger in the laboratory has also been associated with increased distress and aggression in children (Cummings et al., 1985). In sum, there is impressive evidence that frequency is a significant variable to consider in assessing the impact of family environments of conflict.

On the other hand, it is important to guard against an oversimplified view of the impact of the frequency of conflict. Whether and how the frequency of conflict has negative effects is almost certainly influenced by the larger family context. Frequency may interact with other dimensions of family conflict, such as intensity, severity, or destructiveness, as significant or more significant than frequency in accounting for child development outcomes (Jenkins & Smith, 1991).

Frequent parental fighting does not necessarily mean a negative impact on children. Examples of marriages in which the partners fight demonstratively and often but clearly love each other are commonplace. In some families the parents' "fights" may typically be playful or teasing rather than hostile. Some parents may argue as a style of communication, with typically constructive aims and outcomes for themselves and the family. The message or meaning of the parents' conflicts needs to be considered. It is unlikely that the impact on children of a high frequency of constructive disagreements has an impact that is equivalent to the impact of a high frequency of destructive fights.

Modes of Anger Expression

Conflict between individuals is typically thought of as involving verbal exchanges. Children have been found to show distress and other signs of at least temporary disturbance in reaction to verbal conflicts between adults in a long series of studies; such responses have been observed even in infants (Cummings et al., 1981; Cummings et al., 1985). Recent work shows that children are also sensitive to physical aggression and nonverbal expressions of anger.

Interadult Physical Aggression

Interspousal aggression and abuse has been repeatedly associated with the development of behavioral and emotional problems in children (Emery, 1989). Children who witness interparental violence have been shown to be more vulnerable to a wide range of behavior problems (Hershorn & Rosenbaum, 1985; Holden & Ritchie, 1991). For example, psychopathology is approximately four times more likely in children of battered women than in children from nonviolent homes (Jouriles et al., 1989). Interspousal aggression thus clearly adds to the risk associated with exposure to marital discord. In fact, one study reported that interspousal aggression predicted psychopathology in children even after statistically controlling for level of marital discord, suggesting that aggressive behavior between the spouses is an independent predictor of risk for psychopathology in children (Jouriles et al., 1989). Another study found that interspousal violence predicted high rates of behavior problems in children, whereas verbal conflict alone was associated with only low to moderate rates (Fantuzzo et al., 1991).

Observational research supports the contention that interadult aggression is particularly disturbing to children in relation to other modes of anger expression. In the home physical aggression between the parents elicits more distress from children than verbal anger (Cummings et al., 1981). Also, children perceive displays of aggression as more angry than verbal and nonverbal anger expressions (Ballard & Cummings, 1990). Children's emotional responses to interadult aggression are also more negative than to other forms of anger expression (Cummings, Vogel, Cummings, & El-Sheikh, 1989; Cummings, Ballard, & El-Sheikh, 1991).

Nonverbal Anger

Nonverbal expressions of anger are commonplace, but there is surprisingly little research on their impact. What is the impact on children of "dirty looks" and the "silent treatment" between parents? Based on retrospective interviews, one recent study reported no evidence of a relationship nonverbal anger between the parents to child behavior problems (Jenkins & Smith, 1991). However, experimental studies indicate that children are quite sensitive to nonverbal anger expressions between adults. In fact, children report angry or distressed emotions in reaction to nonverbal anger expressions at rates comparable to responses to verbally expressed anger (Ballard & Cummings, 1990; Cummings, Vogel, Cummings, & El-Sheikh, 1989; Cummings, Ballard, & El-Sheikh, 1991).

One possible reason for this apparent inconsistency is that current retrospective methods are insensitive to the occurrence of nonverbal anger and thus fail to detect true associations between nonverbal conflict and children's behavior problems. Nonverbal anger is more subtle and ambiguous than verbal anger and may be considerably more difficult to label and remember. Alternatively, the immediate stressful effects of exposure to nonverbal anger may have no appreciable or lasting effects on children's functioning. However, given the reported amplitude of children's reactions to nonverbal anger expressions in controlled laboratory studies, the likelihood is that nonverbal anger does contribute to the impact of angry home environments on children, particularly when it is chronic and occurs frequently. More work is needed on methodologies to index the cumulative occurrence of nonverbal anger expression in the home.

Intensity

Another dimension of anger expression is intensity. Intuitively, one might expect intense interparental arguments to be more distressing for children than calm, rational disagreements. Consistent with this prediction, one recent analogue study reported that, in relation to low-intensity fights, children reacted to high-intensity conflicts with greater anger, sadness, concern, shame, and helplessness (Grych & Fincham, 1993). Further, children reported more self-blame and reluctance to use direct intervention strategies in response to high-intensity conflicts.

Research based on correlational methodologies has reported links between intense forms of conflict and behavior problems in children (Johnston, Gonzalez, & Campbell, 1987; Wolfe et al., 1985), but these studies do not clearly distinguish between forms of expression of conflict and the intensity of conflict (e.g., physically aggressive fights may more often be rated as intense); hence, this evidence is less conclusive about the effects of intensity as a distinct dimension. A challenge for future research is to distinguish intensity from specific types of anger expression and develop means to assess intensity across the different types.

Content

Thematic content is another aspect of conflict expression. One might suppose that children would be more likely to become distressed when witnessing parental conflicts that are about them (Emery, 1982; Grych & Fincham, 1990), and the evidence is consistent with this prediction. One study reported that, in relation to non-child-related conflicts, children reacted to child-related conflicts with greater shame, self-blame, and fear of being drawn into the conflict (Grych & Fincham, 1993). Another study found that marital fights over child rearing predicted child behavior problems more than either global marital distress or conflicts in areas not related to child rearing (Snyder, Klein, Gdowski, Faulstich, & LaCombe, 1988). Children's emotional difficulties have been related to the incidence of child-rearing disagreements even after controlling statistically for level of marital adjustment and general rate of exposure to marital conflict (Jouriles et al., 1991).

Many questions remain, however, concerning the significance of thematic content to children's coping with background anger. For example, are themes of divorce or threatened separation particularly disturbing? Do children also react to parents' angry discussions of social issues or job-related politics, which are irrelevant to family functioning? What are the effects of parents' use of abusive language as opposed to more careful statements of their feelings for each other? This is another fertile area for future research.

Resolution

Concern has typically focused on how conflict, anger, and hostility is expressed between the parents. However, the ways in which conflicts end, and particularly whether conflicts are resolved, also seem to be important to child outcomes, regardless of how adults express their anger.

A fundamental question is whether children simply attend to how often and how severely parents express anger to each other or whether they perform a more sophisticated assessment of the meaning and implications of parents' conflicts. If children are concerned with the meaning of fights, then whether or not adults resolve their differences should significantly influence the impact of conflict on children.

According to a cognitive–contextual framework for children's coping with background anger (Grych & Fincham, 1990, 1993), the impact of conflict exposure is cognitively mediated and cognitive reappraisals of witnessed conflict can occur after the conflict has ended and information about resolution is presented. Thus, according to this model, one would expect that children's appraisals of interadult conflict would include behavior that occurs after anger expression ends. A related issue is at what age children begin to assess more than simply whether the parents fight.

Observable Resolution

Resolution has repeatedly been shown to reduce the negative impact of background anger on children's emotions and behavior. For example, observational studies have demonstrated that children's aggression and distress in reaction to interadult anger return to baseline levels after the institution of a complete resolution (Cummings, 1987), even among children as young as 2 years of age (Cummings et al., 1985). Children themselves report that their feelings of anger and distress are reduced by a subsequent resolution (Cummings, Vogel, Cummings, & El-Sheikh, 1989). In fact, children's responses to background anger that is followed by a complete resolution are comparable to reactions to entirely friendly interactions (Cummings, Ballard, El-Shiekh, & Lake, 1991; Cummings, Simpson, & Wilson, 1993).

While resolution is often thought of as either present or absent, it is not, in fact, a dichotomous factor; it is more accurately conceptualized along a continuum ranging from no resolution at one extreme to complete resolution at the other. Falling in between these poles are various partial resolutions of conflict. What are the effects on children of variations in the degree of dispute resolution between adults?

Children have been found to be extremely sensitive to even relatively subtle variations in resolution; the relative negativity of children's responses closely corresponds to the degree to which fights were resolved. For example, one study reported that unresolved fights (continued fighting, the silent treatment) elicited more anger from children than partially resolved fights (submission, topic change), which, in turn, resulted in more anger than resolved conflicts (apology, compromise) (Cummings, Ballard, El-Sheikh, & Lake, 1991). Resolved conflicts elicited very little anger.

Resolution Behind Closed Doors

In many families, resolution of parental conflict in the presence of children is not the norm (Vuchinich, Emery, & Cassidy, 1988); parents tend to work things out in private. Do children need to observe resolution to infer its occurrence? How well can children make connections based on relatively sketchy information?

Recently we conducted a study to examine children's responses to resolution "behind closed doors," that is, whether children can infer resolution even when they don't see it (Cummings, Simpson, & Wilson, 1993). We will describe the methodology for this study in some detail because it illustrates a new way of investigating the impact of contextual aspects of anger expression on children. Until recently there were virtually no systematic studies of the effects of specific contexts of interadult conflict on children (Cummings & Cummings, 1988); the development and adoption of new methodologies is a key to advances in this important area.

In our study the children, ranging in age between 5 and 10 years, were presented with a series of videotaped interactions between male and female actors and then asked a series of questions. Rather than being sketchy, hypothetical stories, these videotaped segments were vividly enacted social interactions that were highly engaging for children, who were asked to respond as if they were in the same room as the adults. The aim was to place children in well-defined contexts of exposure to interadult anger that elicit typical reactions, while at the same time minimizing any stress or interpretive confusion associated with repeated exposure to live anger.

Each scenario consisted of a brief conflict followed by one of several endings: no resolution, observed resolution, and two conditions of resolution behind closed doors. For the last two conditions the adults left the room for a period of time following their dispute and then came back and acted friendly toward each other. In the case of implicit unobserved resolution the actors made no mention of their earlier argument, whereas for explicit unobserved resolution they made a brief reference to (but did not describe) an unobserved resolution.

A consistent pattern emerged for children's perceptions of the level of the adults' anger; the anger, sadness, and fear induced in children; and children's perceptions that the problem reflected by the conflict beginning each segment had been worked out. Resolution behind closed doors was a great improvement over no resolution from the children's perspective. Further, children's reactions to unobserved resolution were indistinguishable from responses to observed resolutions. All conditions of resolution were thus highly effective in reducing children's negative responding to interadult conflict. Table 4.1 shows the children's satisfaction levels for the various endings.

While older children made some sharper discriminations between resolved and unresolved anger than did younger children, basic patterns of responding were remarkably similar, regardless of age. Thus, anticipated age differences in the capacity to use relatively sketchy information about resolution were not found. Interestingly, further questioning indicated that children frequently anticipated that adults were in the process of working out their differences when they were out of the room. Thus, expectancies based on past experience with parents in these contexts may have played a role (Grych & Fincham, 1990), enhancing the performance of younger chil-

TABLE 4.1. Children's Satisfaction with Conflict Endings

	5- to 6-year-olds		9- to 10-year-olds	
Condition	Boys	Girls	Boys	Girls
No resolution	2.24	2.03	2.97	2.60
Observed resolution	1.07	1.14	1.07	1.21
Explicit unobserved resolution	1.33	1.00	1.07	1.30
Implicit unobserved resolution	1.21	1.17	1.07	1.07

Scale:
    1 = Problem worked out
    2 = Problem maybe or eventually worked out
    3 = Problem not worked out

dren beyond what might be expected in entirely unfamiliar contexts. Also, an explicit reference to resolution made no difference to children's responding; the temporal cues alone were sufficient for the children to infer resolution.

Finally, reactions using this basic methodology have been shown to be related to children's history of exposure to family conflict. For example, children exposed to more anger in the home show more reactivity to videotaped portrayals of inter-adult conflict (Cummings, Vogel, Cummings, & El-Sheikh, 1989; Hill, Bleichfeld, Brunstetter, Hebert, & Steckler, 1989).

Explained Resolutions

The scenario of adults leaving the room angry and acting friendly upon their return is only one type of cue that a resolution has occurred that children did not observe. (Further, in everyday life this precise temporal sequence of events may not be the one children actually observe.) Sometimes parents directly explain an unobserved resolution to a conflict. A second study reported in Cummings, Simpson, and Wilson (1993) investigated the value of this channel of communication for children. Key questions: Is explanation an adequate substitute for observing resolution, or is it less effective from the child's perspective? Does an explanation following an observed resolution improve on the effects of the observed resolution, or is it superfluous?

In this study children between 5 and 10 years old viewed segments of interadult conflicts that ended with no resolution, observed resolution, friendly interaction, and two contexts of explanation of resolution. For unobserved resolution with explanation the argument was followed by both adults appearing onscreen and one of them explaining how a resolution had been reached. The procedure was the same for observed resolution with explanation except that a resolution between the adults was presented just before the explanation. Explanations consisted of simple, brief narratives describing how the adults had apologized and reached a compromise out of the sight of the children. The explanation scenarios were enacted so that the children could not see that the adults were friendly again (they both simply appeared onscreen together); the children had to relie on what the adults said.

The results presented a relatively consistent picture. Children responded to no resolution most negatively; each of the forms of communicated resolution, observance and explanation, greatly reduced negative responding. In fact, responses to the various resolution conditions and to entirely friendly interactions were comparable. Regardless of age, this basic pattern held across children's various responses to anger, including their perceptions of the adults as angry; their own emotional responses of anger, sadness, and fear; and their perceptions that the problem had been worked out. The results for the last variable are presented in Table 4.2 as an example of this pattern of results.

Explanation thus was another adequate means of communicating an unobserved resolution of interadult disputes. Observing resolution and hearing an explanation of resolution were each entirely effective in reducing children's negative reactions to adults' fights; explanation of an observed resolution was unnecesary and superfluous.

In sum, even relatively young children appear capable of inferring resolution from less complete or less explicit infor-

TABLE 4.2. Children's Satisfaction with Conflict Endings of Resolution and Explanation

Condition	Age group	
	5–6	9–10
No resolution	2.24	2.50
Observed resolution	1.33	1.08
Unobserved resolution with explanation	1.33	1.04
Observed resolution with explanation	1.17	1.04
Friendly interaction	1.02	1.00

Scale:
  1 = Problem worked out
  2 = Problem maybe or eventually worked out
  3 = Problem not worked out

mation than is provided from actually observing the resolution of a dispute. However, the fact that children *can* interpret a variety of types of cues of the occurrence of resolution does not mean that they necessarily *will*. Contextual factors may be critical, such as the length of the interval between adults leaving the room angry and returning together happily in the case of implied resolution behind closed doors. Also, the quality and detail of adults' explanation of the resolution process may affect responding.

Mixed-Message Resolution

There is an important gap in the study of the effects of resolution on children. In most research the affective and content elements of resolution have been presented to children so that they matched—that is, adults who haven't resolved their problems continue to be angry and those who have resolved their differences show positive emotions. What about instances in which affect and content don't match?

In everyday life parents' resolutions may be ambivalent and communicate mixed messages to each other and the rest of the family, which adds another level of complexity to the question of the effects of resolution on children. Conflict endings contain at least two quite different types of information: the actual verbal content or message concerning conflict issues—what the adults actually say to each other—and the valence or tone of the communication—how the adults behave toward each other emotionally, regardless of what they say. These elements may convey significantly different information to the child about the extent to which conflicts are worked out. Is one form of information more important than the other from the child's perspective? Or do children give them more or less equal weighting in evaluating parents' fights?

A recent study has examined this question (Simpson & Cummings, 1993). Following the basic methodology we described in the last two subsections, children were presented with a series of conflicts and conflict endings between a man and woman and then questioned about their perceptions, emotional responses, and likely behaviors as bystanders in the various situations. Following conflicts, the actors engaged in endings that varied in content and emotion. The endings in terms of content were compromise, apology, submission, changing the topic, and continued fighting, and each was presented in a positive and a negative emotional version. Two entirely friendly interactions were also shown.

Children's responses were influenced by both the emotional and content messages of the adults' interactions. Continued fighting was reacted to as most negative and friendly interactions as least negative, and the resolutions (compromise, apology) and partial resolution (submission, topic change) elicited slightly to moderately negative reactions, depending on the affective content of the endings. Negative emotional endings increased the negativity of children's responding. Reactions to changing the topic were typically most affected by the emotional valence of the ending, whereas responses to submission were typically least affected by emotion. Changing the topic elicited quite negative responses when expressed with negative emotion. Responses concerning children's appraisals of whether the problem had been worked out are shown in Table 4.3.

TABLE 4.3. Children's Satisfaction with Conflict Endings

	Age group	
Condition	5–7	9–12
Compromise, positive affect	1.07	1.15
Compromise, negative affect	1.36	1.33
Apology, positive affect	1.12	1.08
Apology, negative affect	1.36	1.47
Submission, positive affect	1.17	1.26
Submission, negative affect	1.16	1.46
Changing the topic, positive affect	1.26	1.16
Changing the topic, negative affect	1.52	2.00
Continued fighting, positive affect	2.07	2.59
Continued fighting, negative affect	2.38	2.78
Friendly (average)	1.00	1.02

One can see that regardless of the affective valence, when there was continued fighting the problem was not seen as resolved. By comparison, each of the resolutions and partial resolutions were viewed as reflecting progress toward a solution of differences. Positive increments in responding occurred when the emotional tone of the interactions was positive. In fact, when affect was positive the responses to compromise and apology were statistically indistinguishable from reactions to entirely friendly interactions.

In sum, children processed the emotional quality as well as the message content of adults' interactions and resolutions, but the message content generally had greater influence on their responding. The affective content caused reactions to message content to be more positive or more negative, depending on whether the emotional valence of the ending was positive or negative, but it did not fundamentally change children's patterns of reactions.

Concluding the section on resolution, recent studies suggest that children do not just react to the fact of conflict; they assess the overall meaning and message of fights between adults, that is, what conflicts convey about how adults are feeling towards each other and how well they are getting along

(Grych & Fincham, 1990; Grych, Seid, & Fincham, 1992). In other words, children process more than just whether adults fight. They engage in an elaborate appraisal that continues after the argument phase has ended and includes an accounting of the result of the interaction. However, the results to date mostly bear on the constructiveness of resolution from the perspective of reducing negative responding. An important question for future study is whether children learn positive lessons from exposure to resolved conflicts, for example, how to appropriately and successfully handle their own disputes.

Explanation: Responsibility, Blame, Problems

As well as explaining resolutions to conflicts, parents in discordant marriages explain to their children their negative relationships. How children respond to such explanations may be pertinent to what children understand about marital breakups and divorce and how such understanding might be facilitated (Buchanan, Maccoby, & Dornbusch, 1991).

Parents' explanations of their relationship can influence children's attributions of responsibility for the parents' fights. Children sometimes assume the blame for parental conflict (Covell & Abramovitch, 1987; Wallerstein & Blakeslee, 1989). Explanations that absolve children from blame reduce their feelings of fear and responsibility, but explanations imputing children as the cause increase their shame and distress (Grych & Fincham, 1993).

Explanation thus can make things worse for children, rather than better. For example, a parent might explain that they fight because daddy is a bad man and that mommy and daddy doesn't love mommy any more, inducing increased distress and anxiety in children. In a more positive vein, the parent might use explanation as a vehicle to help the child understand that while mommy and daddy don't get along and may someday divorce, they both still very much love their children and always will.

When a marital relationship is chronically and unresolvably negative, it might be especially important that the parents explain that their problems are not the child's fault and that the child is not responsible for them. Children from discordant families are especially prone to taking responsibility for the parents' fights (J. S. Cummings et al., 1989a; O'Brien et al., 1991), and to trying to make things better between the parents (Covell & Abramovitch, 1987; Covell & Miles, 1992). Explanations that absolve children from blame for marital problems may help children cope with these stressful family events.

Family and Social Contexts

The impact of marital conflict is likely to be moderated or mediated by the family context in which it occurs. Good parent–child relationships, parental warmth, lack of criticism, and relatively strict monitoring are related to improved functioning in adolescents from discordant families (Hauser, Vieyra, Jacobson, & Wertlieb, 1985; Rutter, 1980). Benefits may even accrue from exposure to moderate conflict in supportive home environments: A context is provided that challenges children to develop skills to effectively cope with stress without overly taxing children's coping resources (Rutter, 1981).

Moderate family conflict is linked with higher levels of social and cognitive functioning in adolescents (Montemayor, 1983; Niemi, 1988). Emotional expressiveness by parents in normal, middle-class families is positively associated with the quality of children's peer relations (Cassidy, Parke, Butkovsky, & Braungart, 1992). One study (Niemi, 1988) reported that the effects of marital conflict on children were quite different in different family contexts. Marital conflict in the context of familial warmth and communication was associated with optimal adolescent development, whereas conflict in a setting of general familial negativity was linked with psychological problems.

Extrafamilial factors may also influence the effect of marital conflict on children, particularly adolescents. As children reach puberty, their involvement in the family declines, and factors outside the family become more important (Hill, Holm-beck, Marlow, Green, & Lynch, 1985). Peer support can buffer the impact of family stressors on adolescents' self-esteem and functioning (Hoffman, Ushpiz, & Levy-Shiff, 1988; Rutter, 1980).

In sum, the general emotional climate of the family and extrafamilial social contexts influence the impact of family conflict on children. However, differences in patterns of conflict may also be a factor. For example, emotionally expressive parents, or those who provide a supportive emotional climate for children, may be more likely to engage in relatively constructive forms of conflict (e.g., an increased rate of resolved marital conflicts). Patterns of conflict expression and the general emotional climate of the family thus may be interrelated. This is an intriguing question for future research.

SPECIFIC ASPECTS OF CONFLICT AND SPECIFIC OUTCOMES: TOWARD A DEVELOPMENTAL PSYCHOPATHOLOGY OF ANGRY HOMES

At this point it ought to be clear that there is considerable complexity in both the stimulus characteristics of angry environments and the types of reactions and responses to anger stimuli that children show. Research must take these realities into account as they increase our understanding of children's development in angry environments. In order to explain the etiology of children's difficulties, one must also factor in time and development. That is, one must account for how different ways of expressing anger and conflict within families over time cause and contribute to different developmental trajectories in children.

Simply put, the goal for a substantive foundation of knowledge for helping children from angry homes is to advance an understanding of relationships between *specific* dimensions of family discord and *specific* child development outcomes, as mediated by *specific* processes (Cummings & Cummings, 1988; Grych & Fincham, 1990; Rutter, 1981). The study of how children develop mental health problems as a result of exposure to marital discord might be referred to as a *developmental psychopathology of angry home environments*.

Figure 4.1 presents elements that need to be considered between exposure to family stressors, such as background anger, and the development of child outcomes. The starting point is the child's response dispositions as elicited by family stressors, such as background anger. The fundamental expression at a process-oriented level of children's risk for adaptive versus maladaptive outcomes are their coping styles, which have relative stability over time and organize multiple emotional, cognitive, and physiological elements of response (Cummings, 1987; Cummings & Cummings, 1988; El-Sheikh et al., 1989). Coping styles, in turn, emerge as a function of children's repeated reactions to anger and the action of certain processes and mechanisms (e.g., induced arousal and resulting dysregulation of emotion and behavior) on their functioning. Some children, as a function of these various influences, are more at risk for conduct disorders, problem aggression, and other externalizing syndromes, whereas others are more at risk for anxiety, withdrawal, depression, and other internalizing syndromes.

One avenue toward developing this model of the effects of family conflict on children is to link exposure to specific types of conflict with specific response processes in children and, in turn, relate specific response processes with clinically significant child outcomes. A number of studies have demonstrated relations between specific elements of conflict expression and specific behavioral and affective response patterns.

For example, interparental physical aggression in the home is positively associated with increased distress responding in children (Cummings, Vogel, Cummings, & El-Sheikh, 1989; J. S. Cummings et al., 1989a) and increased intervention in parental disputes (Barnett, Pittman, Ragan, & Salus, 1980; Christopoulos et al., 1987; J. S. Cummings et al., 1989a;

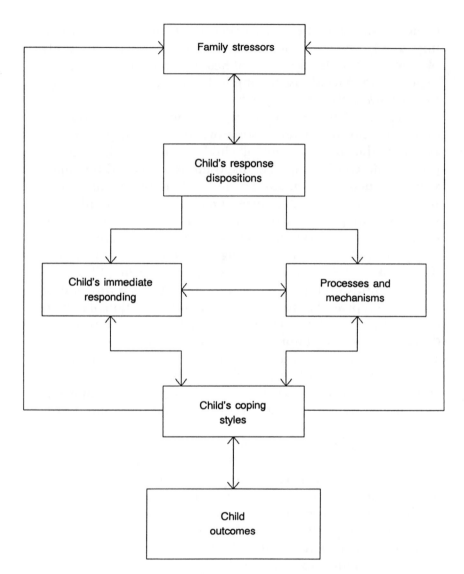

FIGURE 4.1. A conceptualization of the effects of family conflict.

O'Brien et al., 1991). Relations between marital dissatisfaction and heightened distress responding have also been reported (J. S. Cummings et al., 1989a). On the other hand, several studies have failed to find relations between verbal conflict tactics and altered reactivity to anger (E. M. Cummings, Vogel, Cummings, & El-Sheikh, 1989; J. S. Cummings et al., 1989a).

Physical aggression in other family subsystems, such as the parent–child relationship, may also affect response dispositions to anger. One study reported that physically abused children were more fearful than nonabused children in response to interadult anger (Hennessy et al., in press). Another found that physically abused boys became more aggressive and involved in helping the parents after exposure to background anger than non-abused boys (Cummings, Hennessy, Rabideau, & Cicchetti, in press).

Important gaps concern the cumulative effects of exposure to nonverbal anger and the moderating effect over time of the resolution of disputes in the home. Notably, until the development of analogue procedures for studying nonverbal anger and resolution in the laboratory, these processes were seldom considered as relating to the impact of anger on children. Recent experimental findings suggest that these contexts of anger expression are quite significant.

Another important question is whether specific patterns of responding to adults' angry behavior are linked with behavior problems in children. For example, the responses of aggressive children to anger are different than the responses of nonaggressive children. This is of particular interest because aggressiveness and conduct disorder are the problems most frequently linked with angry home environments, as we said in Chapter 1. One study reported that aggressive toddlers showed the greatest increase in aggression toward a same-age peer following exposure to anger between adults (Cummings, Iannotti, & Zahn-Waxler, 1985a). In another study children with behavior problems were more distressed than other children by exposure to background anger (Cummings, Vogel, Cummings, & El-Sheikh, 1989). A third study (Klaczynski &

Cummings, 1989) found that school-age boys classified by their teachers as aggressive were the most aroused by background anger, based on children's self-reports of distress, behavioral impulses, felt emotions, and emotionality in response to anger.

Other at-risk samples also show differences in responding to anger. For example, children of depressed parents are at greater risk for various forms of dysfunction, and increased exposure to marital discord may contribute to their greater risk for behavior problems (Downey & Coyne, 1990). One study (Zahn-Waxler, Cummings, McKnew, & Radke-Yarrow, 1984) found that toddlers of bipolar depressed parents were more likely than toddlers of nondepressed parents to show affective dysregulation as a result of exposure to adults' anger. This is a compelling finding given the very young age of the children and the known risk for affective disregulation in the face of stress associated with bipolar depression. A more recent study reported that dysregulated aggression among 2-year-old children of depressed parents associated with exposure to background anger predicted greater psychiatric difficulties at age 6 (Zahn-Waxler, Iannotti, Cummings, & Denham, 1990).

Children of parents with essential hypertension (EH) are known to be at risk for this disorder, which is thought to relate, in part, to environmental patterns of anger expression and regulation. A recent study of children of EH parents found that sons of EH parents had greater systolic blood pressure reactivity to background anger than sons of normotensive (NT) parents (Ballard, Cummings, & Larkin, 1993). Further, EH family histories did *not* predict behavioral or emotional reactivity to background anger, which was specifically related to parental conflict histories and anger expression in the home. An intriguing notion that follows from these results is that children's areas of vulnerability to exposure to family anger are related to *specific* familial histories and backgrounds.

Finally, alcoholic homes are often characterized by heightened anger, which may contribute to the risk status of children of alcoholic parents (West & Prinz, 1987). A recent study (Ballard & Cummings, 1990) reported that children of alcoholic parents more often wanted to intervene in the disputes of angry adult actors than the children of nonalcoholic parents, particularly by means of indirect involvements designed to make the adults feel better (e.g., cleaning the house, bringing the adults a drink); they were not more likely to suggest direct mediation strategies. Thus, these children were sensitized to solving adults' problems but wary of direct involvements, which in alcoholic homes might well get out of control.

Little is known about response processes mediating relations between marital discord and disorders of withdrawal, anxiety, or other internalizing syndromes (Emery, 1982; Grych & Fincham, 1990). The problem may be one of methodology: Despite the fact that some questionnaires provide for assessing internalizing problems, parents may not be adequate observers of less overt but significant forms of these problems, such as withdrawn behavior, sadness, and anxiety (Compas & Phares, 1991).

In sum, there is an emerging picture of processes mediating relations between specific expressions of family conflict and specific child outcomes. However, marital conflict is not the only influence on children's development; one must also take into account the broader family system of influences on children. Accordingly, in Chapter 5 we will explore interrelations between exposure to conflict and other significant aspects of family functioning.

SUMMARY

There is an emerging, research-based foundation for drawing conclusions about how different aspects of marital conflict affect children. Children are particularly disturbed by conflicts that include physical aggression. The impact of nonverbal expressions of anger on children may be underestimated, and there is a need for parents and others to be more aware of the sensitivity of children to these expressions. The early age at which children are sensitive to conflict and can make inferences based on relatively sketchy information are other noteworthy findings. Children benefit from observing the resolution of conflict and comprehend the occurrence of resolution through a variety of channels of communication.

With the current focus on negative outcomes, it is important to put the occurrence of conflict within families in perspective. Conflicts are surely a normal part of life and may sometimes be necessary for working out important issues concerning marital or family functioning. Exposure to interspousal conflicts may have benefits for children, depending on how conflicts are enacted, how often they occur, and how they are typically ended. The exploration of the constructive effects of exposure to conflict is just beginning. While conflicts followed by resolution induce less negative reactions in children than conflicts that are not resolved, little is known of the specific lessons children learn about resolution styles or optimal social behavior and functioning from "positive" conflicts.

CHAPTER 5

Interparental Conflict
and the Family

Conflict affects children in the context of the family, not in isolation. The impact of exposure to conflict may be modified by the family context, and patterns of conflict expression may magnify or minimize other family influences. Accounting for the effects of interparental conflict on the family requires consideration of more than simply children's experiences of exposure to the parents' fights.

Marital conflict may have indirect as well as direct effects on children. For example, parental fighting is associated with increased hostility between parents and children (Fauber & Long, 1991; Jouriles et al., 1991). By preoccupying the parents, interparental conflict may decrease their sensitivity to their children's needs and signals (Emery, 1982). Such changes in parent–child relations undermine the security of parent–child attachments (Ainsworth et al., 1978; Bowlby, 1973).

On the other hand, parents in conflict may nonetheless maintain good relations with children, remaining responsive to their welfare. In such instances positive parent–child relations help buffer children from the negative effects of marital discord (Emery, 1982). Children with secure attachments are better able to regulate their emotions and behavior when faced with family stresses (Cassidy, 1993; Dix, 1991; Kobak & Sceery, 1988).

Thus, while the parents' patterns of constructive or destructive fighting is important, child outcomes in discordant families ultimately depend on the broad pattern of family functioning. In this chapter we examine the impact of other family systems on children and the relation between interparental conflict and other family systems. One purpose is to present a broader view of child and family relations than is obtained by focusing only on interparental conflict. A particular concern is relations between interparental conflict and general patterns of discord within families.

The marital relationship is just one of several family systems that have significant impact on children's development within families. The parent–child relationship is likely to be of particular importance to child outcomes (Baumrind, 1966; Sears, Maccoby, & Levine, 1957). In this chapter we will consider two important qualities of parent–child relations that are known to significantly affect child development: the parents' styles of interacting and disciplining children, which are called parenting practices, and the quality of the emotional relationship or bond between parents and children, which is called parent–child attachment. These are related but distinct characteristics of parent–child relations (Marvin & Stewart, 1990; Speltz, 1990). We will also consider how children's own characteristics affect their development within families. Recent work suggests that different children may develop in quite different ways even in the same family (Plomin, 1989).

In this chapter we consider how marital conflict can contribute to family dysfunction and thereby affect children's risk for the development of behavior problems. However, while we focus on dysfunction within families, it should be remembered that positive parent–child relations make highly positive and constructive contributions to children's development, and that this may remain the case even when aspects of the marital relationship are dysfunctional.

A way of thinking about family influences on children's development is shown in Figure 5.1. Our assumption is not

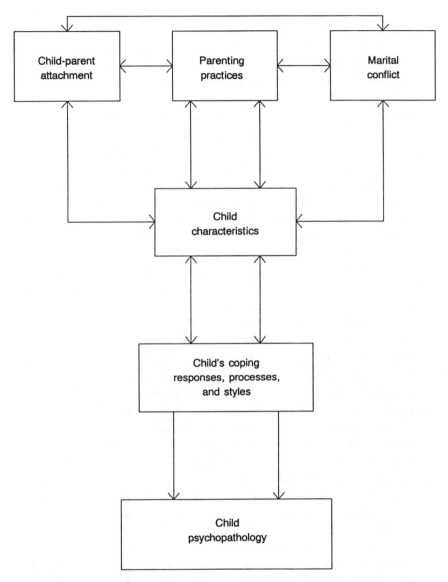

FIGURE 5.1. Family factors and processes underlying relations between family discord and child psychopathology.

that family influences lead directly to positive or negative developmental outcomes but that they mediate or moderate changes in children's coping responses, processes, and styles (Cummings & Cummings, 1988). These changes occur as a function of the accumulating effects of day-to-day exposure to family events and children's reactions to these events. The residue or results of these everyday interactions are gradual changes in children's ways of functioning—changes in children's coping patterns (Cummings & El-Sheikh, 1991).

Some children in some family environments develop dysfunctionally and may be classified as having significant psychopathology (e.g., highly aggressive behavior patterns). Children's behavior problems probably reflect the development of maladaptive coping patterns. For example, aggressive children show greater emotional arousal and aggressiveness than other children in response to background anger (Cummings & Zahn-Waxler, 1992), which might be considered an example of a maladaptive coping pattern.

The identification of the precise coping processes and patterns that lead to desirable and undesirable outcomes among children is an important issue. This level of analysis is often neglected in the traditional focus on "outcomes" in the form of diagnostic labels or scores. However, there is increasing recognition that understanding at a process level ultimately is an important key to a profound understanding of child and family functioning (Garmezy & Rutter, 1983) and, in particular, of the development of psychopathology in children (Cicchetti, 1984; Sroufe & Rutter, 1984). It is not enough to know that child development is altered by discordant processes within the family; one must also know *how* and *why* it is altered.

Figure 5.1 does not include all of the important or potentially important family influences on child development, for example, siblings. Children's brothers and sisters may influence many aspects of their development (Dunn & McGuire, 1992), including the impact of marital conflict. Siblings may try to buffer each other from the stress of exposure to background anger. One recent study found that when siblings were exposed to background anger they exchanged more smiles and played together more altruistically than unrelated children (Cummings & Smith, in press). On the other hand, problems between siblings can increase as a result of marital discord (Brody, Stoneman, & Burke, 1987; Brody, Stoneman, McCoy, & Forehand, 1992).

In sum, this chapter considers how various family systems affect children and interrelations between marital discord and other family systems. An emphasis throughout is identifying the processes and mechanisms that mediate the effects of family discord on children.

INTERPARENTAL CONFLICT

Marital conflict can be considered both a cause and a product of problems within the larger family system (Cummings & Cummings, 1988; Rutter, 1979; Steger & Kotler, 1979). Marital conflict has been associated with childhood psychopathology (see Chapter 1). Furthermore, within dysfunctional families marital discord is an important, if not the primary, predictor of psychological problems in children (Downey & Coyne, 1990; Rutter et al., 1974).

We treat the effects of interadult conflict on children in earlier chapters. The issue here is the processes and mechanisms through which interadult conflict affects children, that is the *why* behind relations between marital conflict and child outcomes.

Negative Reinforcement

Responses by children that reduce the deleterious effects of interparental conflict can be maintained through negative reinforcement (Patterson, 1982). For example, children may interrupt interparental conflicts by misbehaving (e.g., becoming aggressive, crying). Such responses are adaptive in the short run because they distract the parents from their argument to a less serious discipline problem. However, if these behaviors stop the parents' aversive fighting—that is, negative reinforcement occurs—the likelihood that the child will repeat the behaviors in subsequent aversive situations is increased (Emery, 1989). As the negative reinforcement is repeated over and over, the child may show increasingly strong, persistent aversive behaviors in these contexts, contributing to risk for broader patterns of behavior problems.

Arousal and Dysregulation

The arousal induced in children by interparental conflict reduces children's capacity to regulate their own emotions and behavior, at least in the short term. Chronic exposure to interadult conflict is associated with an increase in children's behavioral reactivity in response to background anger and an increase in negative expectations about the future course of adults' conflicts (El-Sheikh & Cummings, 1993; Grych & Fincham, 1990).

Psychological energy and resources are needed to generate and maintain a state of arousal. High, persistent levels of arousal eventually deplete an individual's resources for coping (Cohen & Wills, 1985). The arousal required to respond to chronic interparental conflict competes for resources required to modulate emotions and behavior in other contexts (Cummings & Cummings, 1988). As resources are depleted, a reduction in the quality of children's functioning within and outside of the family may occur.

Repeated exposure to emotionally arousing events intensifies responding (Zillmann, 1983). Thus, repeated exposure to marital conflict energizes or intensifies negative expressions by children, including aggressivness (Cummings & Zahn-Waxler, 1992).

In sum, histories of exposure to background anger may affect children's functioning through arousal-related mechanisms that generally deplete resources for coping with stress and intensify negative responding. Notably, high arousal has also been shown to interfere with the regulation of social and emotional behavior in nonfamily contexts, for example, in relations with peers (Fabes & Eisenberg, 1992a, 1992b).

Modeling Processes

Exposure to interparental conflicts may increase behavior problems in children through modeling (Emery, 1982; Grych & Fincham, 1990; Hetherington & Martin, 1979). Simple imitation (Bandura & Walters, 1963) or the acquisition of "scripts," that is, general strategies for aggressive behavior from observing the parents (Bandura, 1973, 1986) could occur. Further, children's inhibitions about hostile behavior may be reduced by observing angry parents. If the parents as authority figures engage in aggressive behaviors, children become less inhibited because they assume that it is acceptable. While little support for the precise imitation of angry adult models has been found (Cummings et al., 1981, 1985), other modeling-related processes may operate.

MARITAL CONFLICT AND PARENTING

As illustrated in Figure 5.1, parenting and child-rearing practices affect children's development. Like interparental conflict, dysfunctional parenting practices interact with other family and child characteristics in influencing children's development. A family systems perspective is clearly pertinent to understanding the role of dysfunctional parenting practices in contributing to discordant family environments.

Some parenting practices, such as inconsistent discipline, are linked to general disturbances in family functioning (Burgess & Conger, 1978; Lorber, Felton, & Reid, 1984). Problems in parenting are associated with family disorganization, enmeshment and overdependency between family members, marital conflict, and poor family problem-solving strategies

(Loeber & Dishion, 1984; Trickett, Aber, Carlson, & Cicchetti, 1991).

Parenting impairments may be a primary stressor in adverse family environments (Hetherington, 1989; Maccoby & Martin, 1983) and also an outcome of family stress (Belsky, 1980, 1984). Thus family disturbances, such as marital conflict, that increase the parents' arousal and negativity may, inhibit the parents' rational cognitive processes and regulatory abilities (Vasta, 1982). Behavioral dysregulation in the parents, hypersensitivity to negative child behaviors, and increased aggression toward children may result.

Maladaptive child-rearing practices can exacerbate conflict within the family (Patterson, 1986; Patterson & Dishion, 1988). Hostility in parenting and marital relations are interrelated (Jouriles et al., 1989; Wolfe, 1987). There may also be "sleeper effects." For example, parental depression or dysphoria may decrease aversive family interactions in the short term but increase family conflict in the long run (Hops et al., 1987).

Research identifies two elements of dysfunctional parenting: (1) emotional negativity in parenting, and (2) problems in child management. Below, the impact of these dimesions of parenting are considered.

Emotional Negativity in Parenting

Emotional negativity in parenting is linked with children's negative responses and outcomes (Patterson, 1982; Baumrind, 1966; Toth, Manly, & Cicchetti, 1992). Parental passivity, unresponsiveness, and withdrawal are associated with negative child outcomes (Burgess & Conger, 1978; Garbarino, 1989). For example, maternal negativity, intrusiveness, and withdrawal in interactions with children have been shown to elicit anger, reduced activity, dysphoria, and social withdrawal, even in children as young as 3 years of age (Cohn & Campbell, 1992; Cohn & Tronick, 1989; Field, Healy, Goldstein, & Guthertz, 1990). Depressive behaviors in children may occur after prolonged exposure to such interactions (Cohn, Campbell, Matias, & Hoptkins, 1990). In young children a lack of interest in the surrounding environment is observed (Ainsworth, 1979; Bell & Ainsworth, 1972).

Global assessments of the emotional rejection of the child by the parent are linked with both internalizing and externalizing problems. However, two distinct forms of parental emotional rejection can be distinguished: (1) overt hostility toward the child and (2) withdrawal and neglect of the child. The former is most closely linked with childhood problems of aggression and acting out (Hetherington et al., 1992; Olweus, 1980; Wolfe, 1985), and the latter with internalizing problems such as social withdrawal and anxiety (Denham, 1989; Petit & Bates, 1989). Children may model the insensitive styles of their parents. Thus, depressive symptomotology may reflect children emulating their parents' dysphoria, withdrawal, and unresponsiveness (Cicchetti & White, 1988; Field, 1992). Aggression may be due to the vicarious acquisition of the hostile styles of parents (Eron, Monroe, Walder, & Huesmann, 1974; Bandura, 1986).

Insensitive parenting also induces negative arousal (Field, 1987; Tronick, 1989). Short bouts of distress and anger are an initial reaction (Cohn & Tronick, 1983, 1989). Prolonged exposure may sensitize children's arousal systems, making regulation of arousal more difficult (Kopp, 1982). Arousal regulation difficulties are associated with children's aggression (Cummings & Zahn-Waxler, 1992).

Withdrawal from the social environment is another strategy for coping with insensitive parenting. Social withdrawal successfully dampens arousal systems, but it is linked to unresponsiveness, withdrawal, and other internalizing symptomatology in children (Field, 1987, 1992).

Problems in Child Management

Parents use various strategies to discipline and monitor their children. A general finding is that well-adjusted children are monitored fairly closely and experience consistent discipline and authoritative parenting. Many children with behavior problems are subject to inconsistent or lax discipline, coercive or power-assertive control techniques, and authoritarian parenting (Dishion, 1990; Loeber & Dishion, 1984).

Distressed families are often characterized by ineffective child management (Garbarino, Sebes, & Schellenbach, 1984; Patterson, 1982). Parental stress and conflict, preoccupation with their own problems, and lethargy increase parental child management problems (Holden & Ritchie, 1991; Webster-Stratton, 1990). Parental psychopathology (Capaldi & Patterson, 1991) and low socioeconomic status or lack of education about child development (Erickson, Egeland, & Pianta, 1989; Zigler & Hall, 1989) are linked with impaired child management.

The parent's behavioral contingencies or "rules of the game" may inadvertantly reward children's noncompliance and aggression (Patterson, 1982). For example, lax monitoring means that parents cannot effectively deliver consequences for children's misbehavior. Inconsistent discipline creates an intermittent reinforcement schedule (that is, sometimes punishment, sometimes reward for the same behavior) that increases the persistence of undesirable behaviors (Lorber, Felton, & Reid, 1984).

Power-assertive behaviors by parents may create a coercive cycle that provides incentives for misbehavior. The parents may inadvertently use negative reinforcement during episodes of child misbehavior (Patterson, 1982). This typically occurs in escalating, negative exchanges between parents and children. As the child becomes increasingly negative, the distressed parent acts in a positive or neutral manner as a means of escaping additional stress associated with aversive interactions. However, escaping the negative interaction reinforces the child's misbehavior. The result is the negative reinforcement both of the child's aversive behavior that preceded that parental submission and of the parents giving in to the misbehavior. Consequently, in future conflicts the parent is predisposed to submit to the child and the child inclined to exhibit more aversive and antisocial behavior (Patterson, Capaldi, & Bank, 1990).

Power-assertive techniques by parents are also highly arousing for children. Pairing an arousal-inducing stimulus with a negative provocation increases children's disposition to become highly aroused and aggressive in subsequent situations (Zillmann, 1983). Thus, with repeated experience, negative, emotionally arousing parent–child interactions exacerbate children's difficulties with arousal regulation, increasing the risk for behavior problems (Cummings & Zahn-Waxler, 1992).

MARITAL CONFLICT AND ATTACHMENT

Another important category of family influences on child development is the quality of parent–child attachment (see Figure 5.1). Attachment refers to the emotional bond between parent and child, which typically forms in the first year (Ainsworth et al., 1978; Bowlby, 1969). This emotional bond is not fleeting or transient but continues over time, with the quality of attachment also tending to be stable over time (Waters, 1978). Attachment is an important predictor of children's early socioemotional development (Bretherton, 1985).

Attachment research indicates that the quality of the emotional relationship between parents and children is as important to children's development as the strategies and techniques parents use in the relationship (Speltz, 1990). Like other family influences, attachment does not stand alone. The quality of parent–child attachment interacts with other family systems in affecting children's development (Cicchetti, Cummings, Greenberg, & Marvin, 1990; Marvin & Stewart, 1990). For example, parenting is more effective when attachments are secure (Londerville & Main, 1981), and the child's temperament may figure in attachment relationships (Vaughn et al., 1992).

Insecure attachment has been linked with family dysfunction (Belsky, Rovine, & Fish, 1989; Stevenson-Hinde, 1990), including marital conflict (Howes & Markman, 1989). For example, one recent study reported that insecure attachment was associated with a lack of family cohesion ($r = .53$) and low levels of family adaptability ($r = .57$) (Bretherton, Ridgeway, & Cassidy, 1990). Another study found that changes in the security of infant–parent attachments in the second year were related to changes in the family (Egeland & Farber, 1984). Secure infants exposed to family disruption developed more insecure attachments, whereas insecure infants experiencing reduced family discord developed more secure attachments. Parental negativity and insensitivity has been associated with the development of insecure attachment relationships (Ainsworth et al., 1978; Egeland & Sroufe, 1981; Sroufe & Fleeson, 1986).

Dimensions of Attachment

The three main patterns of attachment are secure, insecure–avoidant, and insecure–ambivalent/resistant; very insecure patterns have also been identified, particularly among children from abusing families or families with parental psychopathology (Cicchetti, 1987; Crittenden, 1988; Main & Hesse, 1990; Main & Solomon, 1990; Radke-Yarrow, Cummings, Kuczynski, & Chapman, 1985). A key function of attachment is provision of a sense of security for children, especially in times of stress (Bowlby, 1969; Sroufe & Waters, 1977). Secure attachment fosters behavioral exploration and emotional regulation in children.

Secure attachment is associated with parental responsivity and emotional acceptance of the child (Ainsworth et al., 1978). Securely attached children show less pervasive anxiety and distress than insecurely attached children (e.g., Grossman, Grossman, Spangler, Suess, & Unzer, 1985), and they function more optimally in a wide variety of social domains and contexts (Erickson, Sroufe, & Egeland, 1985; Schneider-Rosen & Cicchetti, 1984; Sroufe, Fox, & Pancake, 1983).

Insecure attachment may reflect a means of coping with dysfunctional family interaction styles (Cummings & El-Sheikh, 1991; Greenberg & Speltz, 1988). For example, repeated rejection by parents is linked with insecure–avoidant attachment (Egeland & Farber, 1984; Lamb, 1987; Sroufe, 1985). In this context avoidance can be seen as serving an adaptive function by limiting the child's involvement with a rejecting parent (Bates & Bayles, 1988; Cassidy & Kobak, 1988; Kobak & Sceery, 1988).

Insecure–ambivalent/resistant attachments have been found to result from disorganized, inattentive parenting and are characterized in children by dependency behaviors toward the parent (e.g., clinging) and expressions of anger. These can be seen as adaptive responses to spousal conflict: Negativity and dependency by children may interrupt and distract parents from spousal conflicts (Cicchetti et al., 1990). Alternatively, the enmeshed nature of this type of attachment may satisfy the anxious emotional needs of a parent whose spouse is disengaged and withdrawn (Byng-Hall, 1990; Stevenson-Hinde, 1990).

While often adaptive within the context of current family systems, insecure attachments are clearly maladaptive in other contexts and are associated with problems of emotional dysregulation (Kobak & Sceery, 1988; Sroufe, 1983), oversensitivity to stress (Lewis, Feiring, McGuffog, & Jaskir, 1984; Sroufe & Fleeson, 1986), and interpersonal relationship problems (Kobak & Sceery, 1988; Erickson et al., 1985; Pastor, 1981). Both externalizing problems (Bates & Bayles, 1988; Cohn, 1990; Speltz, Greenberg, & Deklyen, 1990) and internalizing disorders (Kobak, Sudler, & Gamble, 1991; Lewis et al., 1984; Rubin & Lollis, 1988) in children have been linked with insecure attachment.

Processes and Mechanisms

The influence of the parents' emotional relationship with the child is pervasive, affecting both children's capacity for self-regulation and their social world view.

Arousal and Dysregulation

Children have some of their first experiences with intense affective states—ranging from anger, fear, and anxiety to security, love, and happiness—in the context of the attachment relationship (Ainsworth et al., 1978; Bowlby, 1973). Moreover, the quality and intensity of the emotions experienced by children is affected by the quality of the attachment relationship. Parents of securely attached children are more available and behave more appropriately in helping children regulate their emotions.

Chronic experience with enduring and intense negative emotions may be excessively challenging to the rudimentary capacities of young children to regulate their emotions (Kopp, 1989). Insecurely attached children are more vulnerable to affective and behavioral dysregulation (Cassidy, 1993; Dix, 1991). They harbor more fluctuating and unpredictable affective states, often intensely negative in nature (e.g., excessive anger), than securely attached children (Bowlby, 1988). Consequently, they are more likely to develop emotional and behavior problems (Kobak & Sceery, 1988).

Representations of Relationships

Children develop internal representations of relationships, called internal working models, that can provide a sense of security for them in times of stress. The child's internal working model or representation of the social world of relationships is closely linked to the quality of early attachments. Children's first representations of the self and others develop as a function of the history of parent–child interactions (Bowlby, 1973; Bretherton, 1985; Main, Kaplan, & Cassidy, 1985).

Parental warmth and responsiveness facilitate secure attachment and internal working models characterized by a positive self-concept and confidence in the availability and responsive of others (Cummings & Cicchetti, 1990; Zeanah & Zeanah, 1989). Parental negativity and insensitivity toward children fosters insecure attachment and internal working models of others as unreliable and psychologically unavailable and themselves as unworthy and undeserving of love and affection (Bowlby, 1973; Bretherton, 1985; Sroufe, 1988; Zeanah & Zeanah, 1989). Negative self-cognitions increase the risk for the development of psychopathology, in particular, depression (Cummings & Cicchetti, 1990; Hammen, 1988; Rose & Abramson, 1992).

FAMILY FUNCTIONING AND
THE CHILD'S CHARACTERISTICS

Children are not passive recipients of environmental stimuli. Their various personal characteristics and differences have a major influence on their development.

As illustrated in Figure 5.1, family experiences interact with individual child characteristics and coping processes in influencing child development. It has proven difficult and elusive to measure important dimensions of individual child functioning. One approach is to study individual differences in demographic characteristics, such as age or sex, although age and sex differences must be interpreted with caution, since there can be substantial individual differences within them. Work has also been done on understanding children's cognitive processes and their temperaments.

Demographic Characteristics

Developmental Level/Age

Age differences in cognitive, affective, and behavioral responding to family discord have been reported. The findings do not clearly indicate that any one age group is more vulnerable to family distress and disturbance than the others (see Cummings & Cummings, 1988; Hetherington, 1984; Grych & Fincham, 1990).

Several factors make conclusions about age differences difficult to draw. First, age comparisons are not clearcut because dimensions of functioning change with age. Second, it is difficult to disentangle as causes increasing age and greater exposure to family discord. In comparison to younger children, older children may exhibit greater psychopathology, but it's probably not because they are older but because they have been exposed to family discord over a longer period of time. Finally, children of different ages may be more vulnerable to different types of problems. Age-related vulnerability may not be general but, instead, specific to specific dimensions of psychopathology. While toddlers and preschoolers may deny experiencing feelings of sadness and consider themselves to be predominantly happy, older children seem to consider sadness and happiness as playing roughly equivalent roles in their lives and are increasingly capable of evaluating themselves in a negative manner (Cantwell & Carlson, 1983; Glasberg & Aboud, 1981). Children's internalization of responsibility as they get older may increase their experience of guilt, anxiety, helplessness, and low self-esteem (Harter, 1985; Zahn-Waxler, Kochanska, Krupnick, & McKnew, 1990). Similarly, the capacity to form a global sense of self-worth may allow for stable, negative self-cognitions in older children (Hammen, Burge, & Stansbury, 1990; Harter, 1985).

Sex

Relations between marital discord and behavior problems have more often been reported for boys than for girls (Robins, 1966; Rutter, 1970; West & Farrington, 1973; Wolfe et al., 1985), but the behavior problems of boys are not always found to be greater than those of girls (e.g., Jouriles, Pfiffner, & O'Leary, 1988). As is age, sex is a marker variable for a complex set of processes. Not surprisingly, findings for sex are far from simple (see reviews in Cummings & Cummings, 1988; Grych & Fincham, 1990), but certain patterns are evident.

Among relatively nondistressed families sex differences are often not found (Cummings et al., 1981, 1984; Emery,

1982; Peterson & Zill, 1986). Among clinic-referred children conduct problems are reported more often in boys than in girls (e.g., Emery & O'Leary, 1982; Porter & O'Leary, 1980). Also, when there is family violence (e.g., spouse abuse, child abuse), boys display greater psychological disturbance than girls (Trickett & Susman, 1989; Wolfe et al., 1985). More conduct problems are found among boys when there is divorce (Grych & Fincham, 1992; Hess & Camara, 1979; Hetherington, Cox, & Cox, 1985; Kurdek, 1981), particularly when single mothers obtain custody of the children (Zaslow, 1988, 1989).

Among the explanations for sex differences in behavior problems, some research suggests that males are more susceptible than females to stress, supporting a notion of greater constitutional vulnerability in boys (Eme, 1979; Rutter, 1971; Zaslow & Hayes, 1986). In addition, differences in the socialization of boys and girls may be important (Block, 1983): Parents are more tolerant of misbehavior and aggression in boys (Lytton, 1991), and boys more often become involved in escalating coercive interactions with parents (Maccoby, Snow, & Jacklin, 1984; Patterson, 1982). In comparison to girls, boys are exposed to more parental negativity (Rutter, 1990b), inconsistent discipline (Kurdek, 1986), and psychological insensitivity (Guidubaldi & Perry, 1985). Thus, an interaction between biological vulnerabilities and socialization practices may occur (Lytton, 1991).

Boys' problems may also attract more attention than girls' problems because they are more noticeable. Boys engage in more aggression, misconduct, and impulsivity than girls; girls more often show depression, anxiety, and withdrawal than boys (Block, Block, & Gjerde, 1986; Cohn, 1991; Emery, 1982; Nolen-Hoeksema, 1987). Parents and teachers may simply be more troubled by the destructive behaviors of boys, resulting in an inflated estimate by adults of the incidence of problems in boys in relation to girls (Cummings & Cummings, 1988; Zaslow, 1989).

Sex differences in vulnerability to disorder may change with age. Thus, among divorcing families boys are more susceptible than girls to psychological disturbance in early and middle childhood; problems among boys and girls are of comparable incidence in late childhood and adolescence (Hetherington et al., 1985; Wallerstein, 1985; Zaslow, 1989). A 30-year study of high-risk children found that boys were more vulnerable to psychological problems until adolescence, when girls become more susceptible than boys to psychopathology (Werner, 1989).

Children's Cognitions

Children's cognitions may be a particularly important moderator of relations between family discord and child outcomes (Cummings & Cummings, 1988; Grych & Fincham, 1990). Following is a consideration of some of the types of thinking processes that may be relevant to an understanding of the effects of family disturbance on children.

Views of the Self

Negativity, criticism, and conflict within the parent–child relationship are linked with low self-worth and self-esteem in children (Harter, Marold, & Whitesell, 1992; Jaenicke et al., 1987). Negative views of the self, in turn, predict greater risk for psychopathology in children, for example, depression (Asarnow, Carlson, & Guthrie, 1987; Hammen, 1992; Harter et al., 1992; Panak & Garber, 1992).

Deficiencies in the self-system may interact with other difficulties, resulting in a mutual strengthening of disturbance in children (Cicchetti, 1990; Izard & Schwartz, 1986). Negative self-representations increase vulnerability to stress (Hammen, 1992; Jaenicke et al., 1987) and disrupt the resolution of developmental tasks or challenges (Toth et al., 1992).

Understanding of the Social Environment

Impairment in the processing of social information is associated with family discord (Emery, 1989). For example, maltreated children perceive others' emotions and motives less accurately, display greater insensitivity to others' emotional needs, and show less empathy (Barahal, Waterman, & Martin, 1981). Children from discordant homes selectively attend to and recall negative events, are more likely to blame themselves for negative events, and judge other people as feeling unhappy and angry (Hammen, 1992; Jaenicke et al., 1987; Reichenbach & Masters, 1983). Thus, family discord may sensitize children to negative emotions and increase negative social judgements.

Impairments in thinking processes increase the risk for negative outcomes in children (Dodge, Murphy, & Buchsbaum, 1984; Selman, 1980). For example, self-blame for negative events is a correlate and precursor of depression (Kaslow, Rehm, & Siegel, 1984; Panak & Garber, 1992; Rose & Abramson, in press). Biases toward hostile cognitions are associated with social withdrawal, aggression, peer rejection, and general maladjustment (Dodge, 1980; Dodge & Somberg, 1987; Guerra & Slaby, 1989). Children's low sense of control over marital conflicts are linked to greater physiological reactivity to anger and higher levels of behavior problems (El-Sheikh & Cummings, 1992; Rossman & Rosenberg, 1992).

Some research indicates that impairments in social problem-solving abilities predict negative children's outcomes, regardless of the degree of family stress (Downey & Walker, 1989). Other research suggests that these deficits mediate the impact of family discord (Petit, Dodge, & Brown, 1988).

Children's Temperament

Children with "difficult" temperaments are less sensitive to positive aspects and more susceptible to negative aspects of the social environment; children with "easy" temperaments are more sensitive to the positive aspects and less responsive to the negative aspects (Graham, Rutter, & George, 1973; Rutter & Quinton, 1984; Thompson, 1986). Thus, temperament can either buffer children from family discord or act as a risk factor.

Family functioning may be affected by the child's temperament (see Figure 5.1). Aversive child characteristics tax parental resources, parental caregiving abilities, and the quality of family relationships, increasing disturbance in the larger family system (e.g., Bugental, Mantyla, & Lewis, 1989; Mangelsdorf, Gunnar, Kestenbaum, Lang, & Andreas, 1990). Other correlates of negative child characteristics are parental negativity (Anderson, Lytton, & Romney, 1986; Lee & Bates, 1985), depression (Cutrona & Troutman, 1986; Patterson, 1980), and poor child management techniques (Olweus, 1980). Coercive interactions between the parent and child are increased, making insecure attachment (Belsky et al., 1989; Frodi & Thompson, 1985) and child maladjustment (Petit & Bates, 1984) more likely.

INTERRELATIONS IN FAMILY SUBSYSTEMS

Children's mental health problems do not develop out of parallel and independent disturbances within the family. Rather, disturbances in each family subsystem affects the other subsystems, and broad problems in family functioning are likely to be associated with negative child outcomes. In this section we examine interdependencies as shown by empirical studies of multiple family subsystems, at the level of processes and mechanisms, and in terms of the comorbidity of family stressors.

Empirical Findings

Research on multiple family subsystems strongly supports a model of family subsystems as interrelated. The parents have powerful effects on the child's development, and the marital relationship importantly influences the parents' functioning.

Parenting and Attachment

Parental negativity and psychological unavailability have been shown to be related to insecure attachment in numerous studies (e.g., Ainsworth et al., 1978; Bretherton, 1985, 1990). Particular styles of maladaptive parenting are associated with specific patterns of insecure attachment. Inconsistent, disorganized styles of parenting predict insecure–ambivalent/resistant attachments, whereas parental rejection or physical abuse predict insecure–avoidant attachments (Egeland & Farber, 1984; Grossmann et al., 1985; Main & Cassidy, 1988).

Marital Conflict and Parenting

The stress, frustration, and hopelessness of marital conflict can carry over into parents' interactions with their children (Belsky, 1984; Emery, 1982; Grych & Fincham, 1990). Marital conflict, parenting impairments, and child behavior problems have been shown to be interrelated (Holden & Ritchie, 1991; Jouriles et al., 1988; Fauber et al., 1990). There is increasing evidence that negative changes in parent–child relations due to marital conflict are an important pathway through which family discord contributes to psychopathology in children (Christensen & Margolin, 1988; Crockenberg & Covey, 1991; Fauber et al., 1990).

Marital conflict may influence emotional negativity in parenting more than child management practices. All 13 of the studies surveyed by Davies and Cummings (1993) provided evidence that marital conflict increased emotional negativity in parenting, whereas only 3 out of 5 supported relations between marital conflict and child management problems, and one of these assessments of child management clearly had an emotional component. One implication is that the emotional climate in the home is contagious, moving across relatively permeable boundaries between the various family subsystems.

Marital Conflict and Attachment

Marital conflict may negatively affect attachment by increasing the negativity of parent–child interactions (Marvin & Stewart, 1990) or by decreasing parental involvement and emotional availability. Maritally distressed parents sometimes rely on their children for the emotional support, dependency, and nurturance they do not find in the marital relationship (Stevenson-Hinde, 1990). These added demands on children increase insecurity (Byng-Hall, 1990) and enmeshment (Buchanan et al., 1991; Carlson, Cicchetti, Barnett, & Braunwald, 1989). The negativity of conflict may cause parents to seek affection in other family relations. Children may be pressured to ally with one parent against the other (Johnston et al., 1987; Vuchinich et al., 1988). The undue burdens of these alliances and relational disturbances contributes to the risk of childhood difficulties (e.g., Lewis et al., 1984; Sroufe, 1983), especially withdrawal, anxiety, and dysphoria (Schwarz, 1979).

Several studies indicate relations between marital conflict and insecure parent–child attachment. One study reported that high marital conflict when children were 1 year of age predicted insecure attachment at age 3 (Howes & Markman, 1989). Increases in marital conflict during the first 9 months (Isabella & Belsky, 1985), or even prenatally (Cox & Owen, 1993), are linked to insecure attachment at 12 months of age. Relations have also been reported between marital conflict and other indices of the quality of the emotional relationship between parents and children (Camara & Resnick, 1989; Forehand et al., 1991; Kline et al., 1991; Peterson & Zill, 1986).

In sum, destructive conflict has a particular negative impact on emotional relationships within the family.

Processes and Mechanisms

Family subsystems may affect children's development through their action on common processes and mechanisms. Consequently, there is a possibility that joint effects may occur, which could be additive, interactive, or even multiplicative.

Arousal and Dysregulation

As we have seen, family discord can be highly negatively arousing for children. Over time children's arousal systems may become sensitized by exposure to family discord. It makes intuitive sense that the more sources of highly negatively arousing expressions of family discord, the greater the cumulative negative impact on children's capacities to regulate emotions and behavior.

Modeling, Contingencies, and Reinforcement

We have also seen sources of family discord activate learning processes with negative effects on children's functioning. Again, one would assume that when several subsystems within the family affect the same processes of functioning, the cumulative impact is greater than the sum of the parts.

For example, the behavioral contingencies of coercive parenting reinforce child noncompliance and aggressiveness. Child misbehavior or aggressiveness is negatively reinforced when it terminates marital disputes. Lax monitoring and inconsistent discipline permit or even strengthen the performance of negative behaviors by children. Children witnessing marital conflict may model the emotionally insensitive, dysphoric, or hostile behaviors of the parents.

Cognitive Processes

Children's thinking processes may be disrupted by various forms of family dysfunction. Thus, children's representations of the self may develop negatively from negative parenting interactions or insecure emotional relationships. Further, various impairments in social perceptions and attributions and social skills result from exposure to discordant marital interactions. Negative representations may become long-lasting and resistant to change when children incorporate them as internal working models. Again, the more sources of negative influence on cognitive processes, the greater would seem to be the risk for negative outcomes.

The Comorbidity of Family Stressors

A related issue is the comorbidity of family stressors. One possibility is that the presence of two or more stressors has additive effects. If effects are additive, the combined impact of multiple stressors on children's adjustment would be roughly equivalent to the sum of each of the stressors considered in isolation. However, the picture may not be so simple. A combination of two or more psychosocial stressors may potentiate or multiply children's risk for developing psychological problems; that is, two or more simultaneous family stressors may have far larger effects than the sum of the stressors (Hauser, Vieyra, Jacobson, & Wertlieb, 1985; Rutter, 1980, 1981). Research needs to consider the relations between *combinations of specific stressors* and child outcomes, rather than simply the association between child adjustment and the *number of stressors*.

SUMMARY AND CONCLUSION

The impact of marital conflict on children must ultimately be understood in terms of the family system. Parenting practices, parent–child attachment, and the child's own characteristics are among the other important influences within the family system. Marital conflict may have indirect effects on child development by causing significant perturbations in parenting, attachment, and other subsystems. Further, other subsystems may mediate the impact of exposure to marital conflict on children and in some instances may even buffer children from negative outcomes.

In the final analysis, family functioning is likely to be best understood in terms of the specific mechanisms and processes that mediate relations between family events and child outcomes. Multiple family stressors appear to have an impact on children through the sensitization of arousal processes, thereby increasing the disposition to emotional and behavioral dysregulation in response to stress. Processes of modeling and reinforcement and certain cognitive processes also appear important to the impact of family discord.

CHAPTER 6

Methodology and Message

T hus far we have been concerned with where research on families, conflict, and children has been. In the next two chapters we will address implications and future directions. Research methodology, which is integral to each, is the focus of the present chapter.

Our concern in this chapter is not with relatively narrow technical questions of methodology, which can be trusted to the peer review process and more specialized methodology texts. Rather, our interest is in the scope and range of methods used in the study of family conflict. A central thesis is that methodological diversity and creativity are a key to substantial new advances and the continuing vigor of this field of study.

Knowledge must be considered in the context of the methods used to generate it. Outside technical journals, scientific information is sometimes presented as if it were "objective" and somehow "standing apart" from method. In fact, any meaningful message that can be derived from psychological research is inevitably intertwined with the method(s) used to obtain the knowledge.

Methodology has both explicit and implicit influences on understanding. Explicit effects are relatively obvious and have to do with questions of scientific rigor. Implicit influences are less often recognized but may be even more important to the knowledge generated in an area.

For example, methodology implicitly dictates the types of questions that are asked and the sorts of answers that are sought. Thus, if certain questions are not asked, it may be tacitly concluded that a phenomenon is unimportant. If particular responses are not examined, it may be implicitly assumed that they do not occur. Thus, nonquestions and nonfindings may inadvertently have a very significant impact on the direction and contribution of a field of study.

The importance of methodology is demonstrated by several recent shifts in our understanding of family conflict brought about by the introduction of new methods. For some time, for example, it was concluded that boys were more vulnerable than girls to negative outcomes due to exposure to marital discord. However, much of the research basis for this conclusion was derived from the use of a single methodological approach, that is, questionnaire-based assessments of behavior problems among clinic samples. It is important to note that children are typically referred to clinics because of externalizing behaviors—aggression or acting out—that are easily noted, remembered, and attended to by adults. Since boys typically evidence more externalizing problems and girls more internalizing disorders, more boys are referred to clinics, overemphasizing problematic outcomes among boys in relation to girls. With the advent of observation-based methods, which are much more sensitive to distress and withdrawal as reactions to interparental conflict, it is no longer clear whether boys or girls are more vulnerable; a viable alternative hypothesis is simply that they show problematic reactions in different ways (see Chapter 3).

As another example, many of us are aware from our own personal experience of the power of nonverbal anger and the "silent treatment" as expressions of interpersonal discord. Perhaps we had parents who typically expressed displeasure in their marital relations in this way, and we recall the negative, destructive impact of these expressions on our parents' relationship. We may even remember that it disturbed us as children to observe such communications between our parents.

Until recently, questions of whether nonverbal expressions of anger affected marriages and children simply were not asked; the tacit assumption was that hostility in families was either verbal or physical. This can again be traced to methodology: Prevailing questionnaire-based methods were not well-suited for indexing this dimension of conflict expression for a variety of reasons (e.g., nonverbal anger is less often explicitly labeled and remembered as anger), and no reliable instruments for assessing nonverbal anger expressions had been developed. The introduction of other methods, especially observation-based and analogue studies, has begun to change the perspective on nonverbal communications of anger, demonstrating the impact of nonverbal expressions such as withdrawal and the "silent treatment" on both parents and children (see Chapters 2 and 4).

As a final example, the focus of research until recently had been on the frequency of conflict and anger expression. Thus, the questions for research had to do with how much conflict was too much and what types of anger expression were most destructive. Now there is increasing evidence that the relative constructiveness of conflict, in particular, whether and how conflicts are resolved, is also of substantial importance to marital functioning and children's perceptions of interparental conflicts. This broadening of perspective was associated with the introduction of new methods, specifically, observational studies of marital interaction and analogue investigations of children's reactions to specific scenarios of interadult conflict. Thus, once again, advances in methods of study led the way to new conceptualization of family conflict environments. In sum, methodology and message are much more closely associated than is perhaps commonly appreciated.

The new methods have happened to be observational and analogue procedures, but we do not advocate any one method or set of methods as superior to others; each sound methodological approach is likely to make a contribution. Our goal is the development of more new methods so that problems can be approached in a diversity of ways. Methodological diversity reduces the method dependence of findings. "Truth" is more likely to be found at the crossroads of various approaches, that is, the point at which the methods produce converging and mutually supportive findings.

The virtues of diversity would seem obvious, so perhaps some readers are wondering about the strong emphasis. We feel that it is necessary. In our experience, the forces of tradition, conformity, and familiarity commonly reinforce the "standardization" of methodology in an area, at the same time inadvertantly punishing innovation. Oddly, but serving to demonstrate the sometimes greater influence of peer culture over scientific foundation, the state of the art in one discipline may be looked at askance in related fields. Too often the unfortunate outcome is a lack of integration and cross-fertilization among areas that, in fact, ought to have considerable common ground.

We have long been concerned about this issue as it relates to research on families, conflict, and child development, and we have, accordingly, been active in attempting to develop new field, analogue, and experimental methods (Cummings, 1992; Cummings & Cummings, 1988; Cummings & El-Sheikh, 1991; Davies & Cummings, 1993). Research can become sclerotic and lose vitality because of a lack of creativity and/or resistance to innovation in methodology. A danger is that interest in a construct will be lost because old methods fail to create new information and investigators in an area will not consider new methods. A semicomical but not rare event is that a "lost" but powerful basic phenomenon is "rediscovered" some years later, but with all-new terminology and a general reinvention of the conceptual wheel. This is not an efficient way to proceed!

Continuing methodological innovation is thus important. Our aim is to do more than just decry lack of innovation—we want to suggest some directions toward methodological diversity. Accordingly, in the remainder of this chapter we will make and develop a number of suggestions towards more diversity of method in the investigation of family conflict and child development.

The chapter is organized in three parts. First, we describe

the relative uniformity of method that has typified work on family conflict and children until recently. Next, we briefly consider the principles toward greater diversity in method that have guided our own research on the effects of adults' conflicts on children, which we hope will be useful to others as general guides. Finally, we map out specific future directions for research, including directions for the study of discord and the entire family system.

HISTORICAL TRENDS IN METHODOLOGY

For many years the concern of the field was with establishing basic relationships between marital discord and child outcomes, in particular, associations between high rates of marital conflict and increased behavior problems in children. Research findings supporting this association have accumulated since the 1930s (e.g., Baruch & Wilcox, 1944; Hubbard & Adams, 1936; Towle, 1931; Wallace, 1935); anecdotal reports appeared even earlier (Watson, 1925). Relatively broad-based instruments, such as questionnaires, and relatively general analysis strategies, such as tests for correlations, were appropriate for the types of questions asked and the state of knowledge at the time, and these fundamental relationships were firmly demonstrated (see excellent reviews in Emery, 1982; Grych & Fincham, 1990).

However, while methods may be well suited for some purposes, they may not be ideal for others. Thus, correlational field studies were extremely valuable in calling attention to basic relations between family discord and child development, but interpretive problems arose when investigators attempted to go much beyond making relatively general statements. Further, a variety of significant technical and methodological problems often limited the interpretability of retrospective self-report studies (see Cummings & Cummings, 1988, and Emery, 1982, for further discussion and citations). More fundamentally, global analysis is only likely to yield, with any certainty, relatively global information about family processes—but the relations between child and family functioning are complex and multidimensional.

Sometimes questionnaire-based assessments make substantial claims concerning the specificity of measurement. When performed with considerable attention to psychometric and other measurement concerns, such assessments can make a contribution. However, compelling-sounding labeling does not necessarily mean compelling measurement. Simply positing that a self-reported retrospective series of paper-and-pencil items provides a rigorous, detailed assessment of family or child functioning is not cogent; independent validation is needed.

One common approach is to use one questionnaire with one label to validate another with a different label, but this can be a circular exercise and somewhat misleading. Two purportedly independent questionnaires completed by a single parent may, in fact, reflect precisely the same negative perception of family and personal life. Thus, while the questionnaires may be different, they measure essentially the same response. More technically sophisticated approaches may have *utility*, but inevitably any one method has significant limitations in the perspectives on a phenomenon it provides. In the final analysis, additional and new methods are needed to substantially extend the scope of knowledge.

TOWARD DIVERSITY IN METHODOLOGY

Research in children's responses to interadult anger is now concerned with unraveling the underlying processes accounting for relationships between family conflict and child development. We refer to our own approach as a *process-oriented approach* to children's coping with adults' angry behavior (Cummings & Cummings, 1988). Our twin goals are to increase the scientific understanding of children's basic response processes in coping with family discord and to add to the knowledge base concerning the etiology of clinical problems in children of discordant families, thereby laying the foundation for new and more effective preventive efforts, intervention, and treatment.

The following principles characterize the program pattern of our research, which has been presented throughout this book.

1. *Multiple Methods.* Our commitment to multimethod research reflects an assumption that no one method constitutes a royal road to truth. Every methodology has its strengths and weaknesses. Like blind men feeling different parts of an elephant, each may hold an aspect of the truth, but none provides the whole picture. In our own work, if the use of multiple-methods is not feasible in a single study, we do a programmatic series of studies. While we emphasize the use of experimental and observational methodologies because of their relative rigor, our focal concern is to use methods appropriate to the problems being addressed. Scientific questions should lead to a choice of methods; preferred methods should not limit the scientific questions that are asked.

This ideal has lead us in many directions. Mothers were recruited to make diaries of family conflict, since parents could not be expected to fight on cue with observers present. However, since marital conflict styles vary widely, children were brought to the laboratory and exposed to simulated conflicts in order to focus on describing their own personal coping patterns, without regard to environmental provocation. Finally, we have hooked children up to monitors to document their physiological reactions, and have become television producers to learn of their reactions to specific and multiple forms of anger expressions that seldom occur in pure form in the home and cannot be practically presented in their full array by simulators.

2. *Differentiating Anger Expressions.* Anger has long been implicitly assumed to be a homogeneous stimulus in research and clinical work on family conflict. "Anger" may be a single

word, but it is not a single phenomenon (see Chapter 4). There are many different forms of and contexts for anger expression. A key direction of our work is to differentiate critical dimensions of anger expression between adults from the child's perspective.

Parents may argue in many different ways and, as we have shown, effects of marital conflict on children are highly dependent on how parents fight. To illustrate how recently this point first began to be appreciated, before 1980 virtually no systematic data existed on children's responses to specific and different types of anger expressions. There are undoubtedly many avenues and modes of expression of anger that still remain largely unexplored. For example, patterns for communicating anger nonverbally may be quite complex and diverse—and powerful—but are little understood or investigated.

3. *Considering Multiple Responses.* Just as there is no one way to study anger, there is no one response dimension that provides "truth." Children's response processes are most informatively understood by examining the multiplicity of ways and dimensions in which they respond. Putting this principle in historical context, while many of these response dimensions have now been examined, until about a decade ago there was virtually no information on children's responses to interadult anger beyond retrospective report, typically from the mother.

Cases representative of patterns found are illustrative. Kelly is visibly upset by the parents' arguments and tries, unsuccessfully, to mediate the dispute. By contrast, Keith and Suzy apparently ignore their parents angry disagreement, continuing to play. However, afterwards they become very aggressive towards each other. Edie also seems unaffected, but when a friend asks her later why she is so quiet, she volunteers that she hates it when her parents fight. The notable reaction of another child, Paul, is for his blood pressure to increase as the parents argue. Thus, stress may be shown by individual children in very different ways, indicating the importance of investigating many responses.

4. *Individual Styles of Children's Adaptation to Marital Conflict.* Again, no response or set of responses to the psychological phenomenon of marital discord and anger is typical of all children. Clearly there are marked individual differences in responding. But microscopic levels of analysis may not always provide the best characterization and prediction of child outcomes; broader *patterns* evident across multiple response domains may be most informative. Also, while the focus of research is often on group or mean averages, the identification of distinctive patterns of individual adaptation and maladaptation may ultimately prove to be more useful to scientific understanding and clinical application.

For example, John shows an externalizing pattern of adaptation. He feels very aroused by the parents' fighting, but does not show much emotion himself. However, when another child provokes him later by taking a toy, he becomes quite angry and aggressive towards that child. By contrast, Mary displays an internalizing style. She says little when the parents argue, but is visibly distressed. She cleans up the house and does other good deeds, hoping that this will relieve tensions between the parents.

5. *Age and Developmental Continuity and Change.* It makes intuitive sense that children's ways of responding to and coping with marital discord are different at different ages. Interestingly, however, this issue was virtually unstudied even a decade ago (see review in Emery, 1982). It is significant, from both a scientific and a clinical perspective, to understand how response patterns change as children grow older. Relatedly, it is important to begin to delineate developmental courses of continuity and change in responding, especially as these pertain to the development of mental health problems in children.

6. *Dysfunctional and Normal Families.* Studying both normal and dysfunctional families allows for the understanding of more of the outcomes associated with marital and family conflict. Developmentalists have traditionally constrained their work to the study of the normal end of the population

continuum, whereas clinicians have limited their work to the problematic end. Each type of sampling limits and potentially distorts results. Studying response processes across the continuum of family backgrounds and risk groups yields a more general, informative, and potentially useful knowledge base.

Consistent with this theme, research on children's responses to background anger has included "normal samples" and a variety of samples at risk for various problematic outcomes. The samples studied include children of unipolar depressed parents (Zahn-Waxler et al., 1990) and bipolar depressed parents (Zahn-Waxler et al., 1984), children of alcoholic parents (Ballard & Cummings, 1990), physically abused children (Cummings, Hennessy, Rabideau, & Cicchetti, in press; Hennessy et al., in press), aggressive children (Klaczynski & Cummings, 1989), attention-deficient and hyperactive children (Pelham et al., 1991), children of parents with essential hypertension (Ballard et al., 1993), as well as children from families varying widely in marital discord (J. S. Cummings et al., 1989a).

These themes have served in our work to foster diversity of method and approach. We hope that they will be useful to others.

FUTURE DIRECTIONS IN METHODOLOGY

Several emerging themes in research offer the potential to advance process-level understanding of the impact of family discord, that is, the articulation of relations between specific forms of discord (e.g., marital conflict, dysfunctional parenting) and specific child development outcomes within the context of complex family systems. The themes involve a broader view than simply marital conflict; they concern the larger issue of family discord across multiple family subsystems, consistent with the content of Chapter 5.

Specific Family Stressors

Greater specification is needed for all aspects of the family system.

For example, within the parent–child subsystem specific parenting styles may develop out of different family environments, which may, in turn, have differential effects on child development. For example, aversive child behaviors are correlates of parental neglect but not of parental physical abuse (Wolfe, 1985). Other studies report links between parental neglect and child delinquency and associations between parental hostility/rejection and the development of child anxiety or withdrawal (Hetherington & Martin, 1979). In addition, different parenting styles (e.g., neglect, abuse, inconsistency, rejection) have been found to be correlates of and precursors to different parent–child attachment patterns (e.g., resistant, avoidant, secure) (Bates & Bayles, 1988; Lamb, 1987; Sroufe, 1985).

In marital subsystem, disturbances have often been conceptualized globally as marital dissatisfaction. However, indices of general marital satisfaction/dissatisfaction are markers for a variety of more precise relations between specific aspects of marital discord and child development. For example, one study found that interparental disagreements about child rearing were a better predictor of externalizing disorders in children than general marital adjustment (Jouriles et al., 1991). Other studies have demonstrated that children's reactions vary as a function of the content and intensity of parental arguments, the form of anger expression, and the endings of conflicts (e.g., Grych & Fincham, 1993; Cummings et al., 1989; Cummings, Ballard, El-Sheikh, & Lake, 1991).

Increasing the specificity of the assessment of family stressors will undoubtedly lead to greater understanding of specific process relations and mechanisms contributing to the general association between family discord and child adjustment. Thus, this principle should be applied to the study of all aspects of the family system.

Multiple Dimensions of Children's Responses

Measures of child outcome and response should represent the intricate complexities of children's functioning. Two contrasting types of limitations are evident in current assessments of children's responses: an emphasis on the identification of psychopathology based on global "diagnostic" outcomes, which may preclude a sophisticated analysis of the mechanisms and processes underlying children's difficulties; and the overspecialized study of children's responses in separate, independent behavioral domains, which does not provide a perspective on the complete development and functioning of the child.

Consistent with themes advocated by the discipline of developmental psychopathology (Cicchetti, 1984; Sroufe & Rutter, 1984), assessment research should ideally integrate macroanalytic and microanalytic perspectives. The developmental psychopathology approach views behavior and development in terms of interrelated response constellations that together constitute higher-order patterns and forms of functioning (Cicchetti, 1989; Cicchetti, 1990; Cicchetti & Schneider-Rosen, 1986; Izard & Schwartz, 1986). Consequently, assessment is concerned not with single response domains or global diagnostic assessments but with coherent patterns evident across multiple response domains (Cummings & Cummings, 1988).

The study of higher-order coping styles is another approach toward a more complete understanding of the developmental psychology and developmental psychopathology of discordant families (e.g., Cummings, 1987). Such conceptualizations may help to map out adaptive and maladaptive developmental trajectories of children at a process level. Coping styles or patterns may, in fact, prove to be the best predictors of relations between family discord and children's specific developmental outcomes. Unfortunately, few studies have pursued this level of analysis.

Another valuable approach, consistent with the "triple response" mode (Cone, 1979) or "three-systems" method (Lang, 1968), measures several different response domains, including (1) overt socioemotional behavior during and after exposure to stressors, (2) self-reported emotional responses and behavioral impulses, and (3) physiological responses (e.g., heart rate, blood pressure) across the stressor and poststressor periods (e.g., Ballard et al., 1993; El-Sheikh et al., 1989). In addition to contributing to an understanding of interrelations between behavioral systems and higher-order coping styles, this approach to assessment may lead to more valid interpretations of children's response processes to family discord.

For example, one study (Cummings, 1987) found that a significant subgroup of children responded to interadult anger with no overt emotional responses. Based on examination of these data alone, it might have been concluded that these children were not affected by conflict. However, examination of these children's self-reported feelings and thoughts about the conflict revealed that the children in fact experienced high levels of negative emotional arousal. Notably, only a handful of studies in the child development literature reflect this approach.

The approaches of the studies mentioned might be viewed as inductive approaches to the recognition of coping patterns, as opposed to deductive or theory-driven approaches. Given limitations in the knowledge base, deductive models may well be premature; at the least, the apparent promise of inductive approaches merits much more exploration.

Experimental Designs

While the virtues of experimental designs are well documented, experimental research on the effects of family discord on children has been relatively rare, and much other research has relied on correlational methods. An implicit assumption in many correlational studies is that the independent variables cause or least partially contribute to child outcomes (Dodge, 1990). However, even when high correlations are discovered between variables, little can be said with certainty about the direction of causality. The possibility that extraneous and unassessed variables account for relations always exists. As a result, the mechanisms behind the relations, whether biological or environmental, cannot be identified with confidence.

Experimental designs are well suited to identify the direction of specific process relations within discordant families. As an example, Cohn and Tronick (1983) devised a procedure in which mothers simulated insensitive, intrusive styles of parenting in interactions with their infants under controlled circumstances. Infants were found to respond with negative affective expressions to their mothers' behaviors and eventually disengaged from interaction with their mothers. This experimental design thus demonstrated conclusively the effects of mothers' behavior on infants, providing evidence that environmental factors as well as biological or genetic mechanisms contribute to emotional and behavioral dysregulation in infants.

Constellations of Interrelated Family Stressors

Interrelations between family stressors has been documented (see Chapter 5). A challenge for research is to map out more precisely how these constellations of factors affect child outcomes. The strength and directionality of relations between specific dimensions of family stressors are not well understood. Further, similarities and differences in networks of family stressors in various risk samples and contexts need to be explored further.

Notably, recent research suggests that discordant family processes may critically mediate child outcomes in a wide range of risk samples, including families in which there is child maltreatment (Wolfe, 1987; Jouriles et al., 1989), parental psychopathology (Downey & Coyne, 1990), marital discord (Emery, 1982; Grych & Fincham, 1990), parental alcoholism (West & Prinz, 1987), and child behavior problems (Mash &

Johnston, 1990). However, it cannot be assumed that patterns of effects are the same or even similar in different risk samples.

A goal for future research is to systematically examine the *precise* effects of *specific* constellations of family stressors. Various relations between multiple stressors and developmental outcomes in children have been proposed, including additive (Shaw & Emery, 1988), multiplicative (Rutter, 1981, 1990a), mediating (e.g., Emery, Weintraub, & Neale, 1982; Fauber et al., 1990), and vulnerability/protective (e.g., Brown & Harris, 1978; Rutter, 1981, 1990a) models. Recent methodological suggestions and advancements may facilitate the testing of these models, as well as more complex models of reciprocity between family risk factors.

For example, one report (Walker, Downey, & Nightingale, 1989) provides specific suggestions concerning the advantages of specific statistical techniques (e.g., multiple regression analysis) over other approaches (e.g., ANCOVA, MANCOVA) in examining the relationships between concomitant multiple risk factors and child outcomes (also see Biddle & Marlin, 1987). Another promising development is the recent application of structural equation modeling (SEM) techniques in the analyses of data from developmental and family research (Connell, 1987; Connell & Tanaka, 1987). Rather than statistically isolating relations between a specific predictor and outcome, SEM techniques allow for the specific testing of more complex theoretical models involving the relations among multiple cooccurring predictors and developmental outcomes, and direct versus indirect effects of family stressors.

Further, the use of multivariate statistical techniques may strengthen support for notions of causality and reciprocity among variables; although it must also be recognized that certain statistical assumptions and methodological conditions must be met in order to make such claims and that statements of causality can never be gleaned with complete confidence from nonexperimental data (for more information, see *Child Development, 58*(1), 1987; and more specifically, Mulaik, 1987, and Biddle & Marlin, 1987). Finally, longitudinal research (e.g., Belsky et al., 1989) makes an invaluable, unique contribution to an understanding of causal and reciprocal relations among factors within the family.

Family Relationships and Patterns

One reason for the lag of methodology behind theory and clinical reports is the inherent difficulty of conceptualizing relational and systemic constructs. As Minuchin (1985) points out, "The temptation is to go with the established methodology" since systemic constructs add "a complexity greater than the sum of their parts" (p. 294).

However, several recently developed observation-based methodologies offer promise for assessing systems constructs. The variables that can now be indexed include boundary ambiguity, role reversal, family alliances, triadic interactions, and family relations within subsystems (e.g., Arthur, Hops, & Biglan, 1982; Belsky et al., 1989; Buhrmester, Camparo, Christensen, Gonzalez, & Hinshaw, 1992; Emery, Vuchinich, & Cassidy, 1987; Gjerde, Block, & Block, 1989; Vuchinich et al., 1988).

Conceptual and methodological advances are also being made in assessing family relational constructs. In addition to the conventional focus on child and parent behaviors during parent separation and reunion episodes, researchers have broadened their inquiries to include family members' internal working models of relationships (e.g., Bretherton, 1985; Egeland, Jacobvitz, & Sroufe, 1988; Zeanah & Zeanah, 1989), links between family relationships and capacities for emotional regulation (Kobak & Sceery, 1988), and the adaptive functions of different types of relationships (Bates & Bayles, 1988; Cassidy & Kobak, 1988; Crittenden, 1992).

New methods now permit the assessment of attachment across the life span (Cicchetti et al., 1990; Sroufe & Fleeson, 1986); they include measures for preschoolers (Crittenden,

1992), elementary school children (Cassidy, 1988; Main et al., 1985), adolescents (Kobak & Sceery, 1988), and adults (Barnas, Pollina, & Cummings, 1991; Hazan & Shaver, 1990; Main & Goldwyn, 1984). These methods thus offer the promise of studying family relationship patterns across the generations.

Another promising avenue involves the integration of attachment theory within family systems models (Byng-Hall, 1990; Cicchetti et al., 1990; Easterbrooks & Goldberg, 1990; Marvin & Stewart, 1990; Stevenson-Hinde, 1990). Researchers have noted that attachment patterns (e.g., ambivalent, avoidant, secure) appear to reflect broader systemic conceptualizations of relationship patterns (e.g., enmeshed, disengaged, adaptive). Accordingly, it has been suggested that parent–child attachment patterns not only may serve an adaptive function in the parent–child subsystem, but also may be adaptive for the family system as a whole (Byng-Hall, 1990; Marvin & Stewart, 1990; Stevenson-Hinde, 1990). For example, Stevenson-Hinde (1990) argues that ambivalent parent–child attachment styles may serve an immediate, adaptive function by partially satisfying the anxious emotional needs of a parent whose spouse is disengaged or withdrawn.

Age-Related Changes and Developmental Course

Despite the recent empirical efforts to examine age-related changes and developmental trajectories, there remains a paucity of explicitly developmental research in the family discord literature. Research emphasizing development, however, is necessary in order to understand fully how different family environments affect children. It is only through the delineation of specific developmental patterns in children from various risk environments that we can begin to comprehend which pathways and precursors should be considered aberrant and which ought to be considered normative (Cicchetti, Toth, Bush, & Gillespie, 1988; Sroufe & Rutter, 1984).

The importance of age and developmental level is

reflected in the growing body of research on age differences in children's reactions to family discord. For example, findings from cross-sectional studies on children's responses to family conflict document age differences in children's attributions concerning the origins of parental anger (Harter, 1982, 1983; Covell & Abramovitch, 1987, 1988), perceived efficacy of direct intervention strategies in mitigating marital conflict (Covell & Miles, 1992), proposed involvement in family conflict (Covell & Miles, 1992; J. S. Cummings et al., 1989a), perceptions of emotionality in episodes of interpersonal anger (Cummings, Vogel, Cummings, & El-Sheikh, 1989; Cummings, Ballard, & El-Sheikh, 1991), and emotional responses to interadult conflict (Cummings, Vogel, Cummings, & El-Sheikh, 1989).

Longitudinal assessments based on home observations of family interactions provide evidence for developmental trends in children's social–emotional behavior during family conflict (e.g., Cummings, 1987; Cummings et al., 1984). These studies provide a beginning basis for the identification of developmental periods in which children may be particularly sensitive to the effects of family discord.

A related concern is how children from discordant families approach and resolve salient developmental themes. The latter, also referred to as "stage-salient issues," recognizes development as a series of tasks that become focal at a given period and then remain important throughout an individual's lifetime (for more information, see Cicchetti, 1989, 1990; Cicchetti & Aber, 1986; Cicchetti et al., 1988). For example, stage-salient developmental tasks range from homeostatic regulation between birth and 3 months to emotional regulation at 12 to 30 months of age (Cicchetti, 1989; Cicchetti & Schneider-Rosen, 1986). Successful resolution of these tasks may facilitate normal development, whereas unsuccessful resolution places the child at greater risk for maladaptive development.

For example, Zahn-Waxler, Iannotti, Cummings, and Denham (1990) found that toddlers with mentally ill parents had difficulty achieving the salient developmental task of emotional modulation. Consistent with theoretical proposals, unsuccessful resolution of emotional regulation during toddlerhood predicted subsequent behavior problems for school-age children of mentally ill parents.

Buffers and Resilience Factors

Finally, the concern with psychopathological outcomes of children from discordant homes should not cause researchers to overstate the risk, as children often cope effectively with such conditions; nor should it cause investigators to neglect the existence and important role of buffers and resilience factors in even very discordant environments (Garmezy & Masten, 1991). Unfortunately, relatively little work has been directed toward identifying the factors that buffer or protect children against negative effects associated with growing up in discordant families.

Furthermore, much of the research focuses on identifying inherently pleasant or positive environmental factors that reduce risk for child psychopathology, a limited conceptualization of protective factors. Protective factors may also be negative or stressful. In certain forms, negative events may have "steeling" effects that facilitate the development of adaptive coping styles and thus buffer children from the deleterious impact of stressors (Rutter, 1981, 1990a).

Relatedly, Garmezy argues that the concept of "competence" should be added to the "stress and coping" lexicon to emphasize the role of children's own capacities in overcoming experiential threats and challenges (Garmezy & Masten, 1991). Protective factors and buffers may be internal to the child as well as environmental.

Finally, in addition to identifying protective factors and buffers, there is a need for the systematic examination of the mechanisms that might account for the protective nature of these factors. Relatively little work has been done on this topic.

SUMMARY AND CONCLUSIONS

The theme of this chapter is that methodology and method are inextricably interrelated. Further, limitations in method may reduce the knowledge that can be derived from research, particularly when a single approach or type of approach dominates an area. We argue for the value of a diversity of methods and approaches, and we make a number of specific recommendations for future research on the effects of interadult conflict and, more broadly, family discord on children. The goal is to foster increased flexibility in thinking about method and perhaps even to inspire new sorts of research designs or at least significant modifications of traditional designs.

CHAPTER 7

Conclusions, Implications, and Guidelines

The impact of marital and family conflict on children is of more than academic concern. To the extent that conflict creates distress for children and is linked with the development of mental health problems in children, family conflict is of societal concern and constitutes a significant social problem.

A recent article by Barbara Whitehead (1993) in the *Atlantic* drew attention to the negative effects on children of dissolution of families; the article led this issue to be the all-time best seller in this venerable magazine's long history. As David Broder (1993) noted in the *Washington Post*, the impact on children of the breakdown of families is of great concern for many, regardless of their political philosophy or orientation. Undoubtedly, processes associated with family dissolution, including expression of anger and management of conflict, account for many of the negative outcomes for children.

Problems that lead to family dissolution may continue for years after spouses divorce (Wallerstein & Blakeslee, 1989), with problems in conflict management continuing to be central. One recent study (Buchanan et al., 1991) reported that feelings of being caught between the parents among adolescent children of divorce were related to high parental conflict and hostility and low parental cooperation, which, in turn, were linked with poor adjustment outcomes. Documenting the size of the problem, another major study that followed up on divorced families for many years found a nearly 300% greater rate of clinically significant mental health problems in adolescents from divorced homes than in adolescents in the general population (Hetherington, 1993).

In the preceding chapters we reviewed the scientific evidence pertaining to interadult conflict and child outcomes within families. Practical implications for the conduct of family conflict can be gleaned from this review, but the tone is decidedly academic, consistent with our professional identities. Is it enough to put scholarly work in print, or should more be done to make the work accessible?

Views on the proper roles and responsibilities of researchers are changing. There is an increasing sense that while researchers have an obligation to maintain scholarly rigor, they also have some responsibility for making their findings more accessible. For example, a recent piece in the new journal *Applied and Preventive Psychology* decried the gap between research and practice (Beutler et al., 1993). Interestingly, the problem apparently is not that clinicians are unconvinced of the value of scientific research for their practice but that scientific reports in technical journals are inaccessible to most clinicians. Summarizing clinicians' perception of the problem and its solution, Beutler and colleagues state:

> Based on a survey of how practitioners use psychological research, it appears that clinicians believe that research findings are, and have been, important in modifying their practices. However, they tend to get this "research" information more often from popular books, practice-oriented journals, and workshops than from research journals. Hence, information probably is not coming from scientists and may not actually represent state-of-the-art knowledge. We propose that scientists should market their findings through popular articles and books, workshops, and other vehicles of communication valued by practitioners. (p. 53)

Popular advice about how to handle conflict within families often has little foundation and is sometimes potentially destructive, but the results of systematic studies of family discord and child development are not widely known.

This chapter responds to this concern by providing a more accessible overview of information. We are not clinicians and, appropriately, will not offer clinical advice. However, we can translate the accumulated knowledge into a form that summarizes key points, which then can serve as guides for those in applied areas.

Thus, in this last chapter we provide a listing of conclusions concerning family conflict from the children's perspective that we feel can be made at this time. We also offer principles for conflict expression and for conflict resolution. The last section presents guidelines for more systematic efforts to make research findings available, specifically through research-based parent education and prevention programs. In our view this is a particularly promising vehicle for communicating to parents current information about families, conflict, and conflict resolution from the perspective of the child.

CHILDREN'S RESPONSES TO MARITAL ANGER IN A NUTSHELL

The goal of this section is not to introduce new information but rather to synthesize kernels of knowledge and integrate key points of practical import. The earlier chapters of this volume, along with their extensive citations, provide the scientific foundation for what is said here, and they can be consulted by those who are interested. We intend this section to stand alone for those with entirely practical interests or those wishing a quick summary of basic, recent findings on family conflict and children.

Anger Expression and Conflict Are Normal

The angry behavior and conflicts of parents, when extreme, increase the risk for less than optimal socialization of children, particularly the risk for aggression and behavior problems. However, an overly strong focus on pathological outcomes runs the very real risk of promoting a distorted view of the role of anger expression in family life.

Anger is a natural part of life; everyone, including parents, sometimes becomes angry. Conflict may sometimes be necessary to work out important marital and family issues that could cause further and more serious problems if left unattended (Gottman & Krokoff, 1989). Also, the attempts of parents to suppress angry emotional expression may have a negative effect on children; it is questionable whether parents can truly hide anger from children simply by not verbalizing it (Cummings, Vogel, Cummings, & El-Sheikh, 1989).

The overall message of research is that within certain ill-defined bounds exposure to anger between adults is unlikely to create difficulties for children. There is every reason to believe that children can handle normal levels of anger in the home, even though it may be stressful for them while it is going on. Children are competent and relatively sturdy in coping with everyday stressors; they are not nearly as fragile as they are sometimes represented (Garmezy & Masten, 1991).

A general stereotype is that the more parents argue and the more demonstratively they argue, the greater the likelihood of negative outcomes for children. This is too simple a view of conflict expression and is ultimately misleading. It appears quite possible that the parents may argue a lot but still be close and still have a happy marriage, with no ill effects on children. We have heard many anecdotal examples of such marriages from students and colleagues. The grandparents of one of us (Cummings), for example, constantly teased and disagreed with each other over little things, but they had an extremely close marriage that lasted over 50 years. Some partners clearly enjoy a continual, stimulating back-and-forth and do not interpret disagreement as necessarily significant or negative. For others, even a minor expression of disagreement carries with it relatively dramatic negative meaning and interpretation. This raises a question: Is verbal argument in itself an indicator of marital distress?

Our hypothesis at this point is that it is the underlying message of communication, not the mode of expressing it, that is most important, both to marital partners and to their children. Thus, how much people overtly disagree is not critical; it is the negative emotionality and meaning associated with conflict that has destructive impact

In fact, children's observations of parents' anger and conflict may be necessary experiences in their development of adequate coping skills and ability for relating to others. These experiences may teach them a valuable and constructive lessons about human relations: how to handle the inevitable conflicts of life.

Unfortunately, we know relatively little about what constitutes constructive versus destructive conflicts. We have found that resolution is constructive (Cummings, Vogel, Cummings, & El-Sheikh, 1989), but what are other dimensions of constructive conflict? What are the messages and processes through which children learn to cope with and express conflict from observing their parents' conflicts? Finding out more about the positive side of conflict expression in families ought to be a significant goal for future research.

In sum, it would be unfortunate indeed if this book and the literature reviewed were misinterpreted to indicate that parents should never express conflict or hold their angry feelings in. Bases for concern for children depend substantially on how anger is handled during and after arguments, not whether it is expressed, which must be regarded as quite normal.

Children Are Sensitive to Interadult Conflict

While children can cope with most anger expressions effectively, they are also exquisitely sensitive, dicriminating, and reactive to anger expressions by others, especially parents. They seem almost like emotional geiger counters. A common experience for children is to hear parents fighting or talking about emotional family matters as if the children are not there. We both remember many anecdotal experiences of this sort from our childhoods. While children may not obviously signal their awareness, research suggests that they often accurately understand the emotional content of the parents' communications. Children show discriminative and distressed responses to parental anger at an early age—in the first 6 months of life, according to some research (Shred et al., 1991). Parents may well not be aware of the sensitivity of very young children to their marital fights. It is important for the sake of children's health and well-being in families that this awareness become more general. Young children do not speak well, have relatively poor motor skills, and are immature in their thinking processes. Thus, it is easy for parents to underestimate young children's awareness of emotions and relationships within the family.

The distress and disruption induced in children by exposure to interadult and interparental conflicts are documented by a range of different types of responses. While these reactions are sometimes relatively subtle behaviors that may not be noticed by parents involved in disputes, they are readily detected when children's responses are videotaped or their psychophysiological responses (e.g., heart rate and blood pressure) are recorded in research studies. The overall pattern leaves no doubt about the stressful impact of adults' angry expressions.

Commonly reported responses by children to interadult anger in research include facial expressions of distress, gestures and actions indicative of fear and anxiety (e.g., covering the ears, moving out of the room), freezing (a tense, fixed-in-place posture), increased blood pressure and heart rate, and self-reports of angry, sad, or fearful reactions to adults' fights in interviews conducted after fights have ended (Ballard et al., 1993; O'Brien et al., 1991). Older children sometimes make spontaneous comments about their reactions of anger or anxiety about their parents' fights (J. S. Cummings et al., 1989a), and very young children sometimes cry in response to parents' fights (Cummings et al., 1981).

Of even greater concern in terms of implications for the impact of marital discord on children's development is evidence that exposure to parents' fighting negatively affects children's social functioning not just during the fight but for some period of time after the fights have ended. Children may even be drawn into the parents' disputes, making attempts to mediate interparental disagreements by negotiating between the parents. Studies also document children's efforts at making the parents feel better emotionally by comforting the parents or helping the parents complete or otherwise solve the family problems or unfinished tasks that created the conflicts (Cummings et al., 1981; J. S. Cummings et al., 1989a).

Such role reversal is surely an inappropriate activity, especially for relatively young children. It is the role of the parents to comfort and take care of the children, not the other way around. Notably, mediating reactions by children are highly associated with angry home environments; such reactions are relatively infrequent among children from homes characterized by marital satisfaction and harmony. Parents and others ought to be concerned if younger children frequently adopt the role of "parent" vis-à-vis marital conflict; it would appear to be a warning that family conflict is too high.

One should also be concerned about the appearance of aggressive behaviors in children in maritally distressed homes, given the well-established link between marital conflict and children's behavior problems of aggressiveness. It makes sense that if the stimulus for aggression, that is, interparental conflict, occurs frequently, the pattern of action and reaction may contribute significantly to children's development of aggressive behavior. As with intervention in marital disputes, the more often fights occur, the more likely children are to react with aggression. Thus, children do not get used to conflict or accustomed to it; rather they are sensitized to it and as a result become more vulnerable.

Children Respond Differently to Different Levels of Conflict

Interparental conflict and disagreement is normal and an everyday occurrence, but high levels of conflict do increase the risk for mental health problems in children. This has been documented repeatedly in research conducted over many years. On the other hand, general parental of conflict seems to account for only some negative child outcomes. Our hypothesis is that differences between parents in how they handle conflicts—that is, the relative destructiveness of conflict—account for some of the differences not explained by indices of global conflict rates. Do fights escalate to become very intense or include physical abuse? Are conflicts typically resolved or only rarely resolved? How adequately? Are children blamed for conflicts? An important direction for future research is to develop reliable indices of these dimensions of conflict and add them to current assessment batteries.

The relative impact of conflict on broader family functioning also is not often carefully assessed and may well be an important factor accounting for child development outcomes. For example, does interparental conflict interfere with the quality of the emotional relationship or attachment between parents and children? Does discipline break down as a result of marital conflict? Do parents cease to cooperate and agree on how they should discipline children and on what rules they should enforce? What is the impact of marital conflict on sibling relationships? Do siblings help (e.g., see Cummings & Smith, in press) or hinder (e.g., see Brody et al., 1992) each other in their responses to marital conflict? These are also critical issues for future research.

Children from angry home environments are more sensitive than other children to adults' conflicts. For example, children are much more likely to intervene in parental conflicts when they are from angry homes. Similarly, children from angry home environments are more distressed by adults' fights than others and more likely to become aggressive towards others or destructive of property.

Analogue studies provide particularly convincing evidence of close relations between different types of conflict expression (e.g., resolved versus unresolved conflicts; physical versus verbal conflicts) and children's response patterns. Given control over anger expression and the exclusion of extraneous influences (e.g., effects of marital conflicts on parenting), these studies leave little doubt about causal direction: Differences in adults' anger expression affect children's responding in a variety of important ways.

The findings of field, experimental, and analogue studies thus present a consistent picture: The impact of interadult and interparental conflict on children varies as a function of how adults fight. While sensitivity and reactivity to parental anger in children is normal and found at an early age, heightened sensitivity is linked with relatively destructive forms of anger expressions between the parents. Greater reactivity may, in fact, be dysfunctional, since it is associated with long-term negative child development outcomes.

In addition to environmentally induced differences in coping patterns, children appear to have distinct individual differences in their inherent sensitivity to anger in the family environment (Cummings, 1987). The fact that differences between children appear early and remain stable over significant periods of time suggests that temperamental factors play a role in children's sensitivity and reactivity to interparental anger (Cummings et al., 1984; Cummings, Hollenbeck, Iannotti, Radke-Yarrow, & Zahn-Waxler, 1986). Further, since increased sensitivity and reactivity is linked to negative outcomes (Cummings & Zahn-Waxler, 1992), a child's inherited disposition may also figure in their vulnerability to negative long-term outcomes. In other words, some children are biologically more vulnerable to family discord than others.

In sum, both the specific characteristics of an angry environment in the home and children's own vulnerabilities to parental anger as a stressor contribute to children's relative risk for the development of mental health problems.

Children of Different Ages Respond Differently to Conflict

Age differences in responding are a highly important consideration for understanding the impact of family conflict on children and its possible outcomes and sequelae. While the research indicates that children of all ages, from early infancy to late adolescence, respond to angry conflicts between adults as a stressor, there are definite differences in how children of different ages respond to interadult anger. These findings do not permit the conclusion that any one age is more vulnerable than others; it is simply not yet possible to weigh the available evidence in this way.

Very young children most often react to interparental anger by becoming emotionally distressed or angry. Emotional reactions dominate. Thus, they are most likely to cry, and they report more fear responses than older children. Interventions in parents' fights and other types of coping focused on dealing directly with the problem occur but are relatively uncommon. Most often intervention consists of attempts to distract the parents from their conflict. For example, in one of our studies (Cummings et al., 1981) an instance was reported of a 1-year-old urgently calling, "Mommy, mommy," while the parents were fighting in another room. The mother had to break off the argument to see what the child wanted, thereby interrupting the heated exchange. When the mother entered the child's room, the child merely smiled at her.

Research indicates that at about 5 or 6 years of age the tendency of children to try to mediate parental arguments increases markedly (Cummings et al., 1984; J. S. Cummings et al., 1989a). One study suggests that the disposition to mediate may peak at around middle adolescence (Cummings, Ballard, El-Sheikh, & Lake, 1991), but relatively little work has been done on this issue; more research is clearly needed. Further, it is uncertain whether the capacity to intervene, which can translate into greater enmeshment in the parents' conflicts and "growing up too fast," increases or decreases the children's vulnerability or risk for mental health problems.

While children acquire increasing competence in directly intervening in parents' fights as they get older, they also acquire an increasing awareness of the negative implications of these fights for the family and the child's own welfare. For example, older children are better able to understand that extreme conflict between parents may be a forerunner of divorce.

Boys and Girls React Differently to Conflict

Both boys and girls are affected by exposure to parents' fights, but they show it in different ways. Boys tend to act out, for example, by getting angry or aggressive. Girls show their upset by becoming distressed, anxious, or concerned, reactions that are not as noticeable by adults. However, the fact that girls' responses are less salient does not mean that they are any less upset by parents' fighting. There is no firm basis at this time for concluding that either gender is more or less vulnerable to the impact of interparental fighting.

A sometimes misinterpreted reaction that is more typical of girls is the "perfect child" pattern. Children from angry homes may do more than others to take care of parents' welfare or help around the home. While much more research on the meaning of these behaviors is needed, there is reason to believe that they are not desirable for the child in the long run: Some studies report that such behaviors in young children are linked with negative outcomes years later (Block et al., 1981, 1986).

An intriguing recent finding is that, beginning at around the onset of adolescence, girls report more angry feelings than boys do in reaction to interadult conflict and boys report more sad feelings than do girls (Cummings, Ballard, & El-Sheikh, 1991; Cummings, Ballard, El-Sheikh, & Lake, 1991). This appears to be a reversal of the pattern in earlier years. One interpretation is that adolescent girls' anger reflects a greater sense of responsibility for others whereas adolescent boys' sadness reflects a more detached or withdrawn, albeit sympathetic, reaction.

PRINCIPLES FOR ANGER AND CONFLICT EXPRESSION

Several general implications for how parents can fight constructively for the sake of children have emerged from recent research. These implications are useful for practitioners dealing with distressed marriages and families as well as for parents.

Don't Hold Anger In

We sometimes refer to the "silent treatment" as "middle-class anger." We middle-class types tend to think that if we don't say anything, kids won't notice that anything is wrong. But they most definitely do notice and it makes them anxious.

Consider the following example: Bob and Martha had a fight last night and are still angry with each other while sitting at the breakfast table with their children, Billy (age 8) and Annie (age 6). Bob has a section of the newspaper in front of his face, as does Martha. Only slightly lowering the paper, Bob says, "Please pass the milk, Martha," in a curt way after a long silence. Martha moves the milk just within his reach, without lowering her section of the newspaper at all. Another long silence ensues.

Both parents think that they are handling matters in an "adult" fashion and give no thought to the possibility that their children realize that they are angry with each other. In fact, children between 6 and 8 years of age are likely to be both quite tense in this context and very aware of the negative status of the feelings between the parents.

Several recent studies report that nonverbal expressions of anger are as distressing to children as verbally expressed anger (Cummings, Vogel, Cummings, & El-Sheikh, 1989; Cummings, Ballard, & El-Sheikh, 1991). This is an interesting new finding because nonverbal anger has typically been missed as a potential and significant form of anger expression in research.

Chronic nonverbal anger expression could possibly pose even more problems than verbal anger expression over time, especially in the development of anxiety and depression in children. Verbally unarticulated and unexpressed hostility between the parents is a potential ongoing source of stress for children. No resolution of the parents' conflict is possible because the issues are never put on the table. And nonverbal anger expression models for children the holding in of feelings, conflicts, and anxieties, possibly contributing to the risk for the development of internalizing problems.

Don't Go Overboard When Fighting

In the 1970s and early 1980s, a therapists commonly advocated the desirability of fully ventilating anger as releasing and good for all parties. If one spouse had had an affair, the honest thing to do was to tell the other spouse about it. If one didn't like something about the partner, express it fully. Nerf bats were recommended so that the partners could ventilate their hostilities by (safely) hitting each other.

The notion that the expression of aggression is releasing—the catharsis hypothesis—has not fared well in the research literature. Hostility begets hostility. Say hurtful things to your partner and your partner will be hurtful right back. Worse, if you hit the partner at all, you escalate the hostility to a dangerous point, possibly of no return.

Recent work demonstrates that going overboard in marital conflict is destructive not only for marriages but also for children. Intense expressions of anger are more distressing to children than nonintense expressions (Grych & Fincham,

1993), and anger expressions that include physical aggression between the adults are the most distressing of all (Cummings, Vogel, Cummings, & El-Sheikh, 1989).

The message is clear: Partners should at least control their anger expression so that they do not engage in any physical aggression. Physical anger expression is not only the most distressing form of anger expression from the child's immediate perspective, it is the form of anger expression that has most clearly and consistently been linked with the later development of mental health problems in children. If physical anger expression seems likely to occur, methods for stopping anger should be used. For example, some therapists have advocated constructing rules of fighting that make conflicts less arousing and their outcomes more predictable (e.g., Markman & Kraft, 1989).

PRINCIPLES FOR CONFLICT RESOLUTION

One of the most exciting findings of recent years in our view is evidence that resolution greatly reduces children's negative reactions to interadult conflict. This evidence indicates that children respond not just to the frequency and level of conflict between parents but also to the meaning or the message of conflict. The resolution of conflict indicates that the parents' conflictual interactions have been to some extent constructive, and the children respond accordingly.

Do Resolve Fights

In one recent study (Cummings, Vogel, Cummings, & El-Sheikh, 1989) we found that children's responses to fights that were completely resolved were quite different from their responses to fights that were unresolved, even though the amount and extent of conflict expressed was the same. Resolved fights were responded to in a manner indistinguishable from entirely friendly interactions. The same fights not re-solved were reacted to as negative events.

This result brings home the importance of ensuring that conflicts are not simply a venting of grievances but a means of arriving at an ultimate, positive conclusion of differences. Conflicts move towards a constructive product are beneficial for both parents and children.

The Degree of Resolution Matters

Conflicts are resolved along a continuum between "resolved" and "not resolved." One recent study (Cummings, Ballard, El-Sheikh, & Lake, 1991) indicates that children respond to the degree of resolution. In this study children responded to resolved fights (apology, compromise) in a nonnegative way, to partially resolved fights (topic change, submission of one side to the other) in a moderately negative way, and to un-resolved fights (continued open fighting, the "silent treat-ment" as an ending) in a highly negative way. Thus, the extent to which children were distressed and aroused by adults' fights was a direct function of the degree to which fights were re-solved. An important point to note in this study was that dif-ferent endings were electronically added to the same fight so that the extent and nature of fight was exactly the same. Thus, the endings or outcomes entirely accounted for the results.

Degree of resolution may also be reflected in whether the emotional content of a resolution is positive. For example, a parent may express an apology in an angry way or reach a compromise without any enthusiasm. Other recent work (Cummings, Simpson, Pennington, & Wilson, 1993) suggests that the emotional content of resolution matters, but that a resolved fight still elicits a far less negative response than an unresolved fight, regardless of the emotional tone.

In general, an emotionally positive compromise on issues with apologies appears to be the optimal ending from the children's perspective. But research suggests that children perceive as positive any progress towards resolution.

Children Benefit from Resolution Behind Closed Doors

A recent study (Cummings, Simpson, & Wilson, 1993) indicates that children as young as 5 years of age are able to infer resolution of a conflict when conflicting adults leave a room angry and come back some minutes later acting friendly. In fact, children showed the same nonnegative responses to conflicts resolved behind closed doors as to conflicts they saw openly resolved.

This hopeful result suggests that while it may not always be possible to reach a resolution for awhile after a fight or directly in front of children, children benefit from other forms of information about resolution. Thus, it may be fine for parents to deal with the issues when and how they can. Children may, however, need some cues that a resolution has occurred, even if they are only contextual ones (e.g., a clear change in the emotional communications between the parents some time after a fight).

Children Benefit from Adults' Explanations of Their Conflict Resolutions

Sometimes it may not be possible to provide even contextual cues that differences between adults have been worked out. Under these circumstances the parents may consider explaining their resolution to the children.

Recent work suggests that an explanation of resolution is highly effective in reducing children's negative responses to interadult conflict (Cummings, Simpson, & Wilson, 1993). Children as young as 5 years of age benefitted from a brief explanation of unobserved resolution; their reactions were comparable to those to entirely friendly interactions—almost entirely nonnegative.

In sum, resolution appears to act as a "wonder drug" on the children's perceptions of adults' fights, putting the conflict in a relatively positive rather than highly negative light in their eyes. Perhaps it may be well "okay" for parents to freely express their angry feelings verbally as long as they have a constructive goal in mind and move toward eventual resolution.

A limitation that should be noted is that the power of resolution has been systematically examined only in the relatively artificial confines of laboratory experiments. Such studies indicate how children can react, not necessarily how they actually react. Multimethod investigations are necessary to fully explore the impact of dimensions of family conflict, and field studies are a necessary next step in this line of research.

GUIDELINES FOR RESEARCH-BASED PARENT EDUCATION ON MANAGEMENT OF FAMILY CONFLICT

Turning to the theme of this chapter concerning the need to more effectively disseminate pertinent research findings on family conflict and child development to practitioners and parents, it is apparent that simply putting information in journal or book form may not be an optimal strategy for communicating principles and key issues. Other mechanisms and vehicles need to be found to deliver this information to parents more effectively. Over the past two years, we have taken preliminary steps toward the development of a program to educate parents about the management of conflict for the children's sake based on the available research literature. Kelly Simpson has played a key role in the development of these ideas.

The general model is for parents to be presented with information on optimal versus nonoptimal ways to fight via a videotape program, within the context of a research design that allows for tests of the effectiveness of each element or module of the program. To make the learning process "active" rather than "passive," elements such as group discussions and exercises would be included. The plan is to organize the program in content modules, each presenting a specific "message" about familial conflict and the effect of a form of conflict expression on children.

Research supports the effectiveness of parent education programs based on videotapes (Webster-Stratton, 1981; Webster-Stratton, Hollinsworth, & Kolpacoff, 1989; Webster-Stratton, Kolpacoff, & Hollinsworth, 1988). In a program for the videotape-based training of families with conduct-problem children designed to facilitate better parenting skills and management of family and child life, Webster-Stratton and colleagues reported significant positive changes in behavior both at an immediate posttreatment assessment and at a follow-up interview one year later.

Video formats have the following advantages: (1) the capacity for educational program/training procedures to be reliably reproduced in other settings, (2) the cost effectiveness of educating/training couples with a minimum of person-power, (3) the feasibility of the wide dissemination of the materials, and (4) the high levels of consumer satisfaction associated with video formats for parent education purposes. Video formats increase parents' sense of self-efficacy by allowing them control in solving their problems and being responsible for their own treatment (Webster-Stratton et al., 1989). In addition, from an experimental perspective, the use of videotaped lessons allows greater control over exposure conditions, allowing for a more fine-grained determination of which aspects of the program work and which need remediation.

Videos are ideal for the researcher whose intent is to communicate research knowledge and to aid in prevention and intervention but not to engage in therapy. Thus, careful, precise presentations of information can be constructed that are both faithful to the scientific database and far more accessible and vivid than articles or books.

CONCLUSION

This book provides a survey of the evidence on the risk for behavior problems in children exposed to marital discord, conflict processes in distressed and nondistressed marriages, the direct effects of marital conflict on children, and indirect effects of marital conflict on the family system. Directions are suggested for research and methodological innovation to make possible substantial future progress on this topic. The final chapter summarizes the take-home messages of this research. We hope that this volume provides an impetus for directing renewed concern and work at the effect of interadult conflict on children.

References

Ainsworth, M. D. S. (1979). Attachment related to mother–infant interaction. In J. S. Rosenblatt, R. A. Hinde, C. Beer, & M. Busnel (Eds.), *Advances in the study of behavior* (Vol. 9, pp. 1–51). New York: Academic Press.

Ainsworth, M. D. S., Blehar, M. C., Waters, E., & Wall, S. (1978). *Patterns of attachment: A psychological study of the strange situation*. Hillsdale, NJ: Erlbaum.

Amato, P. R., & Keith, B. (1991). Parental divorce and the well-being of children: A meta-analysis. *Psychological Bulletin, 110,* 26–46.

Anderson, K. E., Lytton, H., & Romney, D. M. (1986). Mothers' interactions with normal and conduct disordered boys: Who affects whom? *Developmental Psychology, 22,* 604–609.

Anderson, S. A., Russell, C. S., & Schumm, W. R. (1983). Perceived marital quality and family life-cycle catagaries: A further analysis. *Journal of Marriage and the Family, 45,* 127–139.

Angold, A., & Rutter, M. (1992). Effects of age and pubertal status on depression in a large clinical sample. *Development and Psychopathology, 4,* 5–28.

Armsden, G. C., & Greenberg, M. T. (1987). The inventory of parent and peer attachment: Individual differences and their relationship to psychological well-being in adolescence. *Journal of Youth and Adolescence, 16,* 427–454.

Arthur, J. A., Hops, H., & Biglan, A. (1982). *LIFE (Living in Familial Environments) coding system.* Unpublished manuscript, Oregon Research Institute, Eugene.

Asarnow, J. R., Carlson, G. A., & Guthrie, D. (1987). Coping strategies, self-perception, hopelessness, and perceived family environments in depressed and suicidal children. *Journal of Consulting and Clinical Psychology, 55,* 361–366.

Ballard, M., & Cummings, E. M. (1990). Response to adults' angry behavior in children of alcoholic and non-alcoholic parents. *Journal of Genetic Psychology, 151,* 195–210.

Ballard, M. E., Cummings, E. M., & Larkin, K. (1993). Emotional and cardiovascular responses to adults' angry behavior and to challenging tasks in children of hypertensive and normotensive parents. *Child Development, 64,* 500–515.

Bandura, A. (1973). *Aggression: A social learning approach.* Englewood Cliffs, NJ: Prentice-Hall.

Bandura, A. (1977). *Social learning theory.* Englewood Cliffs, NJ: Prentice-Hall.

Bandura, A. (1986). *Social foundations of thought and action: A social cognitive theory.* Englewood Cliffs, NJ: Prentice-Hall.

Bandura, A., & Walters, R. H. (1963). *Social learning and personality development.* New York: Holt, Rinehart, & Winston.

Barahal, R. M., Waterman, J., Martin, H. P. (1981). The social cognitive development of abused children. *Journal of Consulting and Clinical Psychology, 49,* 508–516.

Barnas, M. V., Pollina, L., & Cummings, E. M. (1991). Life-span attachment: Relations between attachment and socio-emotional functioning in adult women. *Genetic, Social, and General Psychology Monographs, 117,* 175–202.

Barnett, E. R., Pittman, C. B., Ragan, C. K., & Salus, M. K. (1980). *Family violence: Intervention strategies.* Washington, DC: U.S. Department of H.H.S., Publication No. (OHDS) 80–30258.

Baruch, D. W., & Wilcox, J. A. (1944). A study of sex differences in preschool children's adjustment coexistent with interparental tensions. *Journal of Genetic Psychology, 64,* 281–303.

Bates, J. E., & Bayles, K. (1988). Attachment and the development of behavior problems. In J. Belsky & K. Bayles (Eds.), *Clinical implications of attachment* (pp. 253–299). Hillsdale, NJ: Erlbaum.

Baucom, D. H. (1987). Attributions in distressed relations: How can we explain them? In D. Perlman & S. Duck (Eds.), *Intimate relationships: Development, dynamics, and deterioration* (pp. 177–206). Newbury Park, CA: Sage.

Baucom, D. H., Epstein, N., Sayers, S., & Sher, T. G. (1989). The role of cognition in marital relationships: Definitional, methodological, and conceptual issues. *Journal of Consulting and Clinical Psychology, 57*, 31–38.

Baucom, D. H., & Sayers, S. (1989). The behavioral observation of couples: Where have we lagged and what is the next step in the sequence? *Behavioral Assessment, 11*, 149–159.

Baucom, D. H., Sayers, S., & Duhe, A. (1989). Attributional style and attributional patterns among married couples. *Journal of Personality and Social Psychology, 56*, 596–607.

Baucom, D. H., Sayers, S. L., & Sher, T. G. (1990). Supplementing behavioral marital therapy with cognitive restructuring and emotional expressiveness training: An outcome investigation. *Journal of Consulting and Clinical Psychology, 58*, 636–645.

Baumrind, D. (1966). Effects of authoritative parental control on child behavior. *Child Development, 37*, 887–907.

Beach, S. R. H., & Nelson, G. M. (1990). Pursuing research on major psychopathology from a contextual perspective: The example of depression and marital discord. In G. H. Brody & I. E. Sigel (Eds.), *Methods of family research: Biographies of research projects: Vol. 2. Clinical populations* (pp. 227–259). Hillsdale, NJ: Erlbaum.

Bell, R. Q. (1979). Parent, child, and reciprocal influences. *American Psychologist, 34*, 821–826.

Bell, S. M., & Ainsworth, M. D. S. (1972). Infant crying and maternal responsiveness. *Child Development, 43*, 1171–1190.

Bellah, R. N., Madsen, R., Sullivan, W. M., Swidler, A., & Tipton, S. M. (1985). *Habits of the heart: Individualism and commitment in American life.* New York: Harper & Row.

Belsky, J. (1980). Child maltreatment: An ecological integration. *American Psychologist, 35*, 320–335.

Belsky, J. (1984). The determinants of parenting: A process model. *Child Development, 55*, 83–96.

Belsky, J., & Pensky, E. (1988). Marital change across the transition to parenthood. *Marriage and Family Review, 12*, 133–156.

Belsky, J., & Rovine, M. (1990). Patterns of marital change across the transition to parenthood. *Journal of Marriage and the Family, 52*, 5–19.

Belsky, J., Rovine, M., & Fish, M. (1989). The developing family system. In M. R. Gunnar & E. Thelen (Eds.), *The Minnesota Symposium on Child Psychology: Vol. 22. Systems and development* (pp. 119–166). Hillsdale, NJ: Erlbaum.

Belsky, J., Spanier, G. B., & Rovine, B. (1983). Stability and change in marriage across the transition to parenthood. *Journal of Marriage and the Family, 45,* 567–577.

Berkowitz, L. (1983). The experience of anger as a parallel process in the display of impulsive, "angry" aggression. In R. G. Geen & E. I. Donnerstein (Eds.), *Aggression: Vol 2. Theoretical and empirical reviews* (pp. 103–133). New York: Academic Press.

Berkowitz, L. (1989). Frustration-aggression hypothesis: Examination and reformulation. *Psychological Bulletin, 106,* 59–73.

Beutler, L. E., Williams, R. E., & Wakefield, P. J. (1993). Obstacles to disseminating applied psychological science. *Applied and Preventive Psychology, 2,* 53–58.

Biddle, B. J., & Marlin, M. M. (1987). Causality, confirmation, credulity, and structural equation modeling. *Child Development, 58,* 4–17.

Biglan, A., Hops, H., Sherman, L., Friedman, L., Arthur, J., & Osteen, V. (1985). Problem solving interactions of depressed mothers and their spouses. *Behavior Therapy, 16,* 431–451.

Billings, A. (1979). Conflict resolution in distressed and non-distressed married couples. *Journal of Consulting and Clinical Psychology, 47,* 368–376.

Block, J., Block, J. H., & Gjerde, P. J. (1988). Parental functioning and the home environment in families of divorce: Prospective and concurrent analyses. *Journal of the American Academy of Child and Adolescent Psychiatry, 27,* 207–213.

Block, J. H. (1983). Differential premises arising from differential socialization of the sexes: Some conjectures. *Child Development, 54,* 1335–1354.

Block, J. H., Block, J., & Gjerde, P. J. (1986). The personality of children prior to divorce. *Child Development, 57,* 827–840.

Block, J. H., Block, J., & Morrison, A. (1981). Parental agreement–disagreement on child-rearing orientations and gender-related personality correlates in children. *Child Development, 52,* 965–974.

Bowlby, J. (1969). *Attachment and loss: Vol. 1. Attachment.* New York: Basic Books.

Bowlby, J. (1973). *Attachment and loss: Vol. 2. Separation.* New York: Basic Books.

Bowlby, J. (1980). *Attachment and loss: Vol. 3. Loss.* New York: Basic Books.

Bowlby, J. (1988). *A secure base: Parent–child attachment and healthy human development.* New York: Basic Books.

Bradbury, T. N., & Fincham, F. D. (1987). Affect and cognition in close relationships: Towards an integrative model. *Cognition and Emotion, 1,* 59–87.

Bradbury, T. N., & Fincham, F. D. (1988). Individual difference variables in close relationships: A contextual model of marriage as an integrative framework. *Journal of Personality and Social Psychology, 54,* 713–721.

Bradbury, T. N., & Fincham, F. D. (1989). Behavior and satisfaction in marriage: Prospective mediating processes. *Review of Personality and Social Psychology, 10,* 119–143.

Bradbury, T. N., & Fincham, F. D. (1990). Attributions in marriage: Review and critique. *Psychological Bulletin, 107,* 3–33.

Bradbury, T. N., & Fincham, F. D. (1992). Attributions and behavior in marital interaction. *Journal of Personality and Social Psychology, 63,* 613–628.

Bretherton, I. (1985). Attachment theory: Retrospect and prospect. In I. Bretherton & E. Waters (Eds.), Growing points of attachment theory and research. *Monographs of the Society for Research in Child Development, 50* (1–2, Serial No. 209), 167–193.

Bretherton, I. (1990). Communication patterns, internal working models, and the intergenerational transmission of attachment relationships. *Infant Mental Health Journal, 11,* 237–252.

Bretherton, I., Ridgeway, D., & Cassidy, J. (1990). Assessing internal working models of the attachment relationship. In M. T. Greenberg, D. Cicchetti, & E. M. Cummings (Eds.), *Attachment in the preschool years: Theory, research, and intervention* (pp. 273–308). Chicago: University of Chicago Press.

Broder, D. S. (1993, March 24). Quayle: Right on the family. *The Washington Post,* p. 21.

Brody, G. H., Stoneman, Z., & Burke, M. (1987). Family system and individual child correlates of sibling behavior. *American Journal of Orthopsychiatry, 57,* 561–569.

Brody, G. H., Stoneman, Z., McCoy, J. K., & Forehand, R. (1992). Contemporaneous and longitudinal associations of sibling conflict with family relationship assessments and family discussions about sibling problems. *Child Development, 63,* 391–400.

Brown, G., & Harris, T. (1978). *Social origins of depression.* London: Tavistock.

Buchanan, C. M., Maccoby, E. E., & Dornbusch, S. M. (1991). Caught between parents: Adolescents' experience in divorced homes. *Child Development, 62,* 1008–1029.

Bugental, D. B., Mantyla, S. M., & Lewis, J. (1989). Parental attributions as moderators of affective communication to children at risk for physical abuse. In D. Cicchetti & V. Carlson (Eds.), *Child maltreatment: Theory and research on the causes and consequences of child abuse and neglect* (pp. 254–279). New York: Cambridge University Press.

Buhrmester, D., Camparo, L., Christensen, A., Gonzalez, L. S., & Hinshaw, S. P. (1992). Mothers and fathers interacting in dyads and triads with normal and hyperactive sons. *Developmental Psychology, 28,* 500–509.

Burgess, R. L., & Conger, R. D. (1978). Family interaction in abusive, neglectful, and normal families. *Child Development, 49,* 1163–1178.

Byng-Hall, J. (1990). Attachment theory and family therapy: A clinical view. *Infant Mental Health Journal, 11,* 228–236.

Buss, A. H., & Plomin, R. (1975). *A temperament theory of personality development.* New York: Wiley.

Cadoret, R., O'Gorman, T., Heywood, E., & Troughten, E. (1985). Genetic and environmental factors in major depression. *Journal of Affective Disorders, 9,* 155–164.

Camara, K. A., & Resnick, G. (1989). Styles of conflict resolution and cooperation between divorced parents: Effects on child behavior and adjustment. *American Journal of Orthopsychiatry, 59,* 560–575.

Camper, P. M., Jacobson, N. S., Holtzworth-Munroe, A., & Schmaling, K. B. (1988). Causal attributions for interactional behaviors in married couples. *Cognitive Research and Therapy, 12,* 195–209.

Cantwell, D. P., & Carlson, G. A. (1983). Issues in classification. In D. P. Cantwell & G. A. Carlson (Eds.), *Affective disorders in childhood and adolescence* (pp. 19–38). New York: Spectrum.

Capaldi, D. M., & Patterson, G. R. (1991). Relation of parental transitions to boys' adjustment problems: I. A linear hypothesis. II. Mothers at risk for transitions and unskilled parenting. *Developmental Psychology, 27,* 489–504.

Carlson, V., Cicchetti, D., Barnett, D., & Braunwald, K. G. (1989). Finding order in disorganization: Lessons from research on maltreated infants' attachments to their caregivers. In D. Cicchetti & V. Carlson (Eds.), *Child maltreatment: Theory and research on the causes and consequences of child abuse and neglect* (pp. 494–528). New York: Cambridge University Press.

Cassidy, J. (1988). Child–mother attachment and the self at age six. *Child Development, 57,* 331–337.

Cassidy, J. (1993, March). Emotion regulation within attachment relationships. In J. Cassidy & L. Berlin (Chairs), *Attachment and emotions*. Symposium conducted at the meeting of the Society for Research in Child Development, New Orleans, LA.

Cassidy, J., & Kobak, R. R. (1988). Avoidance and its relation to other defensive processes. In J. Belsky & T. Nezworski (Eds.), *Clinical implications of attachment* (pp. 300–323). Hillsdale, NJ: Erlbaum.

Cassidy, J., Parke, R. D., Butkovsky, L., & Braungart, J. M. (1992). Family–peer connections: The roles of emotional expressiveness within the family and children's understanding of emotions. *Child Development, 63,* 603–618.

Chelune, G. J., Waring, E. M., Vosk, B. N., Sultan, F. E., & Ogden, J. K. (1984). Self-disclosure patterns in clinical and nonclinical couples. *Journal of Clinical Psychology, 40,* 213–215.

Chodorow, N. (1978). *The reproduction of mothering: Psychoanalysis and the sociology of gender.* Berkeley, CA: University of California Press.

Christensen, A. (1988). Dysfunctional interaction patterns in couples. In P. Noller & M. A. Fitzpatrick (Eds.), *Perspectives on marital interaction* (pp. 31–52). Clevedon, England: Multilingual Matters.

Christensen, A., & Heavey, C. L. (1990). Gender and social structure in the demand/withdraw pattern of marital conflict. *Journal of Personality and Social Psychology, 59,* 73–81.

Christensen, A., & Margolin, G. (1988). Conflict and alliance in distressed and nondistressed families. In R. A. Hinde & J. Stevenson-Hinde (Eds.), *Relationships within families* (pp. 263–282). New York: Oxford University Press.

Christensen, A., & Nies, D. C. (1980). The Spouse Behavior Observation Checklist: Empirical analysis and critique. *American Journal of Family Therapy, 8,* 69–79.

Christensen, A., & Shenk, J. L. (1991). Communication, conflict, and psychological distance in nondistressed, clinic, and divorcing couples. *Journal of Consulting and Clinical Psychology, 59,* 458–463.

Christopoulos, C., Cohn, D. A., Shaw, D. S., Joyce, S., Sullivan-Hanson, J., Kraft, S., & Emery, R. E. (1987). Children of abused women: I. Adjustment at time of shelter residence. *Journal of Marriage and the Family, 49,* 611–619.

Cicchetti, D. (1984). The emergence of developmental psychopathology. *Child Development, 55,* 1–7.

Cicchetti, D. (1987). Developmental psychopathology in infancy: Illustration from the study of maltreated youngsters. *Journal of Consulting and Clinical Psychology, 55,* 837–845.

Cicchetti, D. (1989). How research on child maltreatment has informed the study of child development: Perspectives from developmental psychopathology. In D. Cicchetti & V. Carlson (Eds.), *Child maltreatment: Theory and research on the causes and consequences of child abuse and neglect* (pp. 377–431). New York: Cambridge University Press.

Cicchetti, D. (1990). An historical perspective on the discipline of developmental psychopathology. In J. Rolf, A. Masten, D. Cicchetti, K. Nuechterlein, & S. Weintraub (Eds.), *Risk and protective factors in the development of psychopathology* (pp. 2–28). New York: Cambridge University Press.

Cicchetti, D., & Aber, J. L. (1986). Early precursors of later depression: An organizational perspective. In L. Lipsitt & C. Rovee-Collier (Eds.), *Advances in infancy* (Vol. 4, pp. 87–137). Norwood, NJ: Ablex.

Cicchetti, D., Cummings, E. M., Greenberg, M. T., & Marvin, R. S. (1990). An organizational perspective on attachment beyond infancy. In M. T. Greenberg, D. Cicchetti, & E. M. Cummings (Eds.), *Attachment in the preschool years: Theory, research, and intervention* (pp. 3–49). Chicago: University of Chicago Press.

Cicchetti, D., & Schneider-Rosen, K. (1986). An organizational approach to childhood depression. In M. Rutter, C. E. Izard, & P. B. Read (Eds.), *Depression in young people: Developmental and clinical perspectives* (pp. 71–134). New York: Guilford Press.

Cicchetti, D., Toth, S., Bush, M., & Gillespie, J. (1988). Stage-salient issues: A transactional model of intervention. *New Directions for Child Development, 39,* 123–145.

Cicchetti, D., & White, J. (1988). Emotional development and affective disorders. In W. Damon (Ed.), *Child development today and tomorrow* (pp. 177–198). San Francisco: Jossey-Bass.

Cohen, S., & Wills, T. A. (1985). Stress, social support, and the buffering hypothesis. *Psychological Bulletin, 98,* 310–357.

Cohn, J. F., & Campbell, S. B. (1992). Influence of maternal depression on infant affect regulation. In D. Cicchetti & S. Toth (Eds.), *Rochester Symposium on Developmental Psychopathology: Vol. 4. A developmental approach to affective disorders.* Rochester, NY: University of Rochester Press.

Cohn, J. F., Campbell, S. B., Matias, R., & Hopkins, J. (1990). Face-to-face interactions of postpartum depressed and non-depressed mother–infant pairs at 2 months. *Developmental Psychology, 26,* 15–23.

Cohn, J., & Tronick, E. (1983). Three-month-old infants' reaction to simulated maternal depression. *Child Development, 54,* 185–190.

Cohn, J. F., & Tronick, E. Z. (1989). Specificity of infants' response to mothers' affective behavior. *Journal of the American Academy of Child and Adolescent Psychiatry, 28,* 242–248.

Cohn, L. D. (1991). Sex differences in the course of personality development: A meta-analysis. *Psychological Bulletin, 109,* 252–266.

Compas, B. E., & Phares, V. (1991). Stress during childhood and adolescence: Sources of risk and vulnerability. In E. M. Cummings, A. L. Green, & K. H. Karraker (Eds.), *Life-span developmental psychology: Perspectives on stress and coping* (pp. 111–129). Hillsdale, NJ: Erlbaum.

Cone, J. D. (1979). Confounded comparisons in triple response mode assessment research. *Behavioral Assessment, 1,* 361–373.

Connell, J. P. (1987). Structural equation modeling and the study of child development: A question of goodness of fit. *Child Development, 58,* 167–175.

Connell, J. P., & Tanaka, J. S. (1987). Introduction to the special section on structural equation modeling. *Child Development, 58,* 2–3.

Covell, K., & Abramovitch, R. (1987). Understanding emotion in the family: Children's and parents' attributions of happiness, sadness, and anger. *Child Development, 58,* 976–984.

Covell, K., & Abramovitch, R. (1988). Children's understanding of maternal anger: Age and source of anger differences. *Merrill-Palmer Quarterly, 34,* 353–368.

Covell, K., & Miles, B. (1992). Children's beliefs about strategies to reduce parental anger. *Child Development, 63,* 381–390.

Cox, M. J. (1985). Progress and continued challenges in understanding the transition to parenthood. *Journal of Family Issues, 6,* 395–408.

Cox, M. J., & Owen, M. T. (1993, March). Marital conflict and conflict negotiation: Effects on infant–mother and infant–father relationships. In M. Cox & J. Brooks-Gunn (Chairs), *Conflict in families: Causes and consequences.* Symposium conducted at the meeting of the Society for Research in Child Development, New Orleans, LA.

Coyne, J. C., Burchill, S. A. L., & Stiles, W. B. (1991). An interactional perspective on depression. In C. R. Snyder & D. O. Forsyth (Eds.), *Handbook of social and clinical psychology: The health perspective* (pp. 327–348). New York: Pergamon.

Crittenden, P. M. (1988). Relationships at risk. In J. Belsky & T. Nezworski (Eds.), *Clinical implications of attachment* (pp. 136–174). Hillsdale, NJ: Erlbaum.

Crittenden, P. M. (1992). Quality of attachment in the preschool years. *Development and Psychopathology, 4,* 209–241.

Crockenberg, S. B., & Covey, S. L. (1991). Marital conflict and externalizing behavior in children. In D. Cicchetti & S. Toth (Eds.), *Rochester Symposium on Developmental Psychopathology: Vol. 3. Research and clinical contributions to a theory of developmental psychopathology.* Rochester, NY: University of Rochester Press.

Cummings, E. M. (1987). Coping with background anger in early childhood. *Child Development, 58,* 976–984.

Cummings, E. M. (1992). Mechanisms mediating relations between marital discord and children's behvaior problems. *West Virginia Journal of Psychological Research and Practice, 1,* 97–104.

Cummings, E. M., Ballard, M., & El-Sheikh, M. (1991). Responses of children and adolescents to interadult anger as a function of gender, age, and mode of expression. *Merrill-Palmer Quarterly, 37,* 543–560.

Cummings, E. M., Ballard, M., El-Sheikh, M., & Lake, M. (1991). Resolution and children's responses to interadult anger. *Developmental Psychology, 27,* 462–470.

Cummings, E. M., & Cicchetti, D. (1990). Toward a transactional model of relations between attachment and depression. In M. T. Greenberg, D. Cicchetti, & E. M. Cummings (Eds.), *Attachment in the preschool years: Theory, research, and intervention* (pp. 339–372). Hillsdale, NJ: Erlbaum.

Cummings, E. M., & Cummings, J. L. (1988). A process-oriented approach to children's coping with adults' angry behavior. *Developmental Review, 8,* 296–321.

Cummings, E. M., & Davies, P. T. (in press). Maternal depression and child development. *Journal of Child Psychology and Psychiatry.*

Cummings, E. M., & El-Sheikh, M. (1991). Children's coping with angry environments: A process-oriented approach. In M. Cummings, A. Greene, & K. Karraker (Eds.), *Life-span developmental psychology: Perspective on stress and coping* (pp. 131–150). Hillsdale, NJ: Erlbaum.

Cummings, E. M., Hennessy, K. D., Rabideau, G. J., & Cicchetti, D. (in press). Coping with anger involving a family member in physically abused and non-abused boys. *Development and Psychopathology.*

Cummings, E. M., Hollenbeck, B., Iannotti, R., Radke-Yarrow, M., & Zahn-Waxler, C. (1986). Early organization of altruism and aggression: Developmental patterns and individual differences. In C. Zahn-Waxler, E. M. Cummings, & R. Iannotti (Eds.), *Altruism and aggression* (pp. 165–188). New York: Cambridge University Press.

Cummings, E. M., Iannotti, R. J., & Zahn-Waxler, C. (1985a). The influence of conflict between adults on the emotions and aggression of young children. *Developmental Psychology, 21,* 495–507.

Cummings, E. M., Iannotti, R. J., & Zahn-Waxler, C. (1985b). Unpublished videotaped laboratory situations.

Cummings, E. M., Iannotti, R. J., & Zahn-Waxler, C. (1989). Aggression between peers in early childhood: Individual continuity and developmental change. *Child Development, 60,* 887–895.

Cummings, E. M., Simpson, K., Pennington, L., & Wilson, A. (1993, March). Fighting constructively: Children's reaction to everyday contexts of interpersonal conflict resolution. In E. M. Cummings (Chair), *Contexts of interparental conflict and child behavior.* Syposium conducted at the meeting of the Society for Research in Child Development, New Orleans, LA.

Cummings, E. M., Simpson, K. S., & Wilson, A. (1993). Children's responses to interadult anger as a function of information about resolution. *Developmental Psychology, 29,* 978–985.

Cummings, E. M., & Smith, D. (in press). The impact of anger between adults on siblings' emotions and social behavior. *Journal of Child Psychology and Psychiatry.*

Cummings, E. M., Vogel, D., Cummings, J. S., & El-Sheikh, M. (1989). Children's responses to different forms of expression of anger between adults. *Child Development, 60,* 1392–1404.

Cummings, E. M., & Zahn-Waxler, C. (1992). Emotions and the socialization of aggression: Adults' angry behavior and children's arousal and aggression. In A. Fraczek & H. Zumkley (Eds.), *Socialization and aggression.* New York and Heidelberg: Springer-Verlag.

Cummings, E. M., Zahn-Waxler, C., & Radke-Yarrow, M. (1981). Young children's responses to expressions of anger and affection by others in the family. *Child Development, 52,* 1274–1282.

Cummings, E. M., Zahn-Waxler, C., & Radke-Yarrow, M. (1984). Developmental changes in children's reactions to anger in the home. *Journal of Child Psychology and Psychiatry, 25,* 63–74.

Cummings, J. S., Pellegrini, D., Notarius, C., & Cummings, E. M. (1989a). Children's responses to angry adult behavior as a function of marital distress and history of interparent hostility. *Child Development, 60,* 1035–1043.

Cummings, J. S., Pellegrini, D., Notarius, C., & Cummings, E. M. (1989b). Unpublished videotaped laboratory situations.

Cutrona, C. E., & Troutman, B. R. (1986). Social support, infant temperament, and parenting self-efficacy: A mediational model of postpartum depression. *Child Development, 57,* 1507–1518.

Davies, P. T., & Cummings, E. M. (1993). *Marital conflict and child adjustment: A process-oriented approach.* Manuscript submitted for publication.

Denham, S. A. (1989). Maternal affect and toddlers' socioemotional competence. *American Journal of Orthopsychiatry, 59,* 368–376.

Dishion, T. J. (1990). The family ecology of boys' peer relations in middle childhood. *Child Development, 61,* 874–892.

Dix, T. (1991). The affective organization of parenting: Adaptive and maladaptive processes. *Psychological Bulletin, 110,* 3–25.

Dodge, K. (1980). Social cognition and children's aggressive behavior. *Child Development, 51,* 162–170.

Dodge, K. (1990). Developmental psychopathology in children of depressed mothers. *Developmental Psychology, 26,* 3–6.

Dodge, K. A., & Frame, C. (1982). Social cognitive biases and deficits in aggressive boys. *Child Development, 53,* 620–635.

Dodge, K. A., Murphy, R. R., & Buchsbaum, K. (1984). The assessment of intention-cue detection skills in children: Implications for developmental psychopathology. *Child Development, 55,* 163–173.

Dodge, K. A., & Somberg, D. R. (1987). Hostile attributional biases among aggressive boys are exacerbated under conditions of threats to the self. *Child Development, 58,* 213–224.

Doherty, W. J. (1981a). Cognitive processes in intimate conflict: I. Extending attribution theory. *American Journal of Family Therapy, 9,* 3–13.

Doherty, W. J. (1981b). Cognitive processes in intimate conflict: II. Efficacy and learned helplessness. *American Journal of Family Therapy, 9,* 35–44.

Doherty, W. J. (1982). Attributional style and negative problem solving in marriage. *Family Relations, 31,* 201–205.

Downey, G., & Coyne, J. C. (1990). Children of depressed parents: An integrative review. *Psychological Bulletin, 108,* 50–76.

Downey, G., & Walker, E. (1989). Social cognition and adjustment in children at risk for psychopathology. *Developmental Psychology, 25,* 835–845.

Dunn, J., & McGuire, S. (1992). Sibling and peer relationships in childhood. *Journal of Child Psychology and Psychiatry, 33,* 67–105.

Easterbrooks, M. A., & Goldberg, W. A. (1990). Security of toddler–parent attachment. In M. T. Greenberg, D. Cicchetti, & E. M. Cummings (Eds.), *Attachment in the preschool years: Theory, research, and intervention* (pp. 221–244). Chicago: University of Chicago Press.

Egeland, B., & Farber, E. (1984). Infant–mother attachment: Factors related to its development and changes over time. *Child Development, 55,* 753–771.

Egeland, B., Jacobvitz, D., & Sroufe, L. A. (1988). Breaking the cycle of abuse. *Child Development, 59,* 1080–1088.

Egeland, B., & Sroufe, L. A. (1981). Developmental sequelae of maltreatment in infancy. *New Directions for Child Development, 11,* 77–92.

Eidelson, R. J., & Epstein, N. (1982). Cognition and relationship maladjustment: Development of a measure of dysfunctional relationship beliefs. *Journal of Consulting and Clinical Psychology, 50,* 715–720.

El-Sheikh, M., & Cummings, E. M. (1992). Perceived control and preschoolers' responses to interadult anger. *International Journal of Behavioral Development, 15,* 207–226.

El-Sheikh, M., & Cummings, E. M. (in press). Children's responses to angry adult behavior as a function of experimentally manipulated histories of exposure to resolved and unresolved anger. *Social Development.*

El-Sheikh, M., & Cummings, E. M. (1993). *Preschoolers' responses to interadult anger: The role of experimentally manipulated exposure to resolved and unresolved arguments.* Manuscript submitted for publication.

El-Sheikh, M., Cummings, E. M., & Goetsch, V. (1989). Coping with adults' angry behavior: Behavioral, physiological, and self-reported responding in preschoolers. *Developmental Psychology, 25,* 490–498.

Eme, R. F. (1979). Sex differences in childhood psychopathology: A review. *Psychological Bulletin, 86,* 574–595.

Emery, R. E. (1982). Interparental conflict and the children of discord and divorce. *Psychological Bulletin, 92,* 310–330.

Emery, R. E. (1988). *Marriage, divorce, and children's adjustment.* Newbury Park, CA: Sage.

Emery, R. E. (1989). Family violence. *American Psychologist, 44,* 321–328.

Emery, R. E., Fincham, F. D., & Cummings, E. M. (1992). Parenting in context: Systemic thinking about parental conflict and its influence on children. *Journal of Consulting and Clinical Psychology, 60,* 909–912.

Emery, R. E., & O'Leary, K. D. (1982). Children's perceptions of marital discord and behavior problems of boys and girls. *Journal of Abnormal Child Psychology, 10,* 11–24.

Emery, R. E., & O'Leary, K. D. (1984). Marital discord and child behavior problems in a nonclinic sample. *Journal of Abnormal Child Psychology, 12,* 411–420.

Emery, R. E., Vuchinich, S., & Cassidy, J. (1987). *Manual for the Third Party Intervention Scoring System (TPICS).* Unpublished manuscript, University of Virginia, Charlottesville.

Emery, R. E., Weintraub, S., & Neale, J. M. (1982). Effects of marital discord on the school behavior of children of schizophrenic, affectively disordered, and normal parents. *Journal of Abnormal Child Psychology, 10,* 215–228.

Epstein, N., & Eidelson, R. J. (1981). Unrealistic beliefs of clinical couples: Their relationship to expectations, goals, and satisfaction. *American Journal of Family Therapy, 9,* 13–22.

Epstein, N., Pretzer, J. L., & Fleming, B. (1987). The role of cognitive appraisal in self-reports of marital communication. *Behavior Therapy, 18,* 51–69.

Erickson, M. F., Egeland, B., & Pianta, R. (1989). The effects of maltreatment on the development of young children. In D. Cicchetti & S. Toth (Eds.), *Child maltreatment: Theory and research on the causes and consequences of child abuse and neglect* (pp. 647–684). Cambridge, England: Cambridge University Press.

Erickson, M. F., Sroufe, L. A., & Egeland, B. (1985). The relationship between quality of attachment and behavior problems in preschool in a high-risk sample. In I. Bretherton & E. Waters (Eds.), Growing points in attachment theory and research. *Monographs of the Society for Research in Child Development, 50* (1–2, Serial No. 209), 147–166.

Eron, L. D., Monroe, M. M., Walder, L. O., & Huesmann, R. (1974). Relation of learning in childhood to psychopathology and aggression in young adulthood. In A. Davids (Ed.), *Childhood personality and psychopathology: Current topics* (pp. 53–88). New York: Wiley.

Fabes, R. A., & Eisenberg, N. (1992a). Young children's coping with interpersonal anger. *Child Development, 63,* 116–128.

Fabes, R. A., & Eisenberg, N. (1992b). Young children's emotional arousal and anger/agressive behaviors. In A. Fraczek & H. Zumkley (Eds.), *Socialization and agression* (pp. 85–101). New York and Heidelberg: Springer-Verlag.

Fantuzzo, J. W., DePaola, L. M., Lambert, L., Martino, T., Anderson, G., & Sutton, S. (1991). Effects of interparental violence on the psychological adjustment and competencies of young children. *Journal of Clinical and Consulting Psychology, 59,* 258–265.

Fauber, R., Forehand, R., Thomas, A. M., & Wierson, M. (1990). A mediational model of the impact of marital conflict on adolescent adjustment in intact and divorced families: The role of disrupted parenting. *Child Development, 61,* 1112–1123.

Fauber, R. L., & Long, N. (1991). Children in context: The role of the family in child psychotherapy. *Journal of Consulting and Clinical Psychology, 59,* 813–820.

Fendrich, M., Warner, V., & Weissman, M. M. (1990). Family risk factors, parental depression, and psychopathology in offspring. *Developmental Psychology, 26,* 40–50.

Field, T. M. (1987). Affective and interactive disturbances in infants. In J. D. Osofsky (Ed.), *Handbook of infant development* (2nd ed., pp. 972–1005). New York: Wiley.

Field, T. (1992). Infants of depressed mothers. *Development and Psychopathology, 4,* 49–66.

Field, T., Healy, B., Goldstein, S., & Guthertz, M. (1990). Behavior-state matching and synchrony in mother–infant interactions of nondepressed vs. depressed dyads. *Developmental Psychology, 26,* 7–14.

Fincham, F. D. (1985). Attribution processes in distressed and non-distressed couples: 2. Responsibility for marital problems. *Journal of Abnormal Psychology, 94,* 183–190.

Fincham, F. D., Beach, S. R., & Baucom, D. H. (1987). Attribution processes in distressed and nondistressed couples: 4. Self–partner attribution differences. *Journal of Personality and Social Psychology, 52,* 739–748.

Fincham, F. D., Beach, S. R., & Nelson, G. (1987). Attribution processes in distressed and nondistressed couples: 3. Causal and responsibility attributions for spouse behavior. *Cognitive Therapy and Research, 11,* 71–86.

Fincham, F. D., & Bradbury, T. N. (1987). The impact of attributions in marriage: A longitudinal analysis. *Journal of Personality and Social Psychology, 53,* 510–517.

Fincham, F. D., & Bradbury, T. N. (1988). The impact of attributions in marriage: An experimental analysis. *Journal of Social and Clinical Psychology, 7,* 122–130.

Fincham, F. D., & O'Leary, K. D. (1983). Causal inferences for spouse behavior in maritally distressed and nondistressed couples. *Journal of Social and Clinical Psychology, 1,* 42–57.

Fitchen, C. S. (1984). See it from my point of view: Videotape and attributions in happy and distressed couples. *Journal of Social and Clinical Psychology, 2,* 125–142.

Floyd, F. J., & Markman, H. J. (1983). Observational biases in spouse interaction: Toward a cognitive behavioral model of marriage. *Journal of Consulting and Clinical Psychology, 51,* 450–457.

Follingstad, D. R., Rutledge, L. L., Berg, B. J., Hause, E. S., & Polek, D. S. (1990). The role of emotional abuse in physically abusive relationships. *Journal of Family Violence, 5,* 107–120.

Forehand, R., Wierson, M., Thomas, A. M., Fauber, R., Armstead, L., Kempton, T., & Long, N. (1991). A short-term longitudinal examination of young adolescent functioning following divorce: The role of family factors. *Journal of Abnormal Child Psychology, 19,* 97–111.

Freed, D. J., & Foster, H. H. (1981). Divorce in the fifty states: An overview. *Family Law Quarterly, 14,* 229–241.

Frodi, A., & Thompson, R. (1985). Infants' affective responses in the Strange Situation: Effects of prematurity and quality of attachment. *Child Development, 56,* 1280–1290.

Gaelick, L., Bodenhausen, G. V., & Wyer, R. S. (1985). Emotional communication in close relationships. *Journal of Personality and Social Psychology, 49,* 1246–1265.

Gantz, J., & Gantz, H. (Producers/Directors). (1985). *Couples arguing* [Film]. Mill Valley, CA: View Film and Video.

Garbarino, J. (1989). Troubled youth, troubled families: The dynamics of adolescent maltreatment. In D. Cicchetti & S. Toth (Eds.), *Child maltreatment: Theory and research on the causes and consequences of child abuse and neglect* (pp. 685–706). Cambridge, England: Cambridge University Press.

Garbarino, J., Sebes, J., & Schellenbach, C. (1984). Families at risk for destructive parent–child relations in adolescence. *Child Development, 55,* 174–183.

Garmezy, N., & Masten, A. S. (1991). The protective role of competence indicators in children at risk. In E. M. Cummings, A. L. Greene, & K. H. Karraker (Eds.), *Life-span developmental psychology: Perspectives on stress and coping* (pp. 151–176). Hillsdale, NJ: Erlbaum.

Garmezy, N., & Rutter, M. (1983). *Stress, coping, and development in children.* New York: McGraw-Hill.

Gassner, S., & Murray, E. J. (1969). Dominance and conflict in the interaction between parents of normal and neurotic children. *Journal of Abnormal Psychology, 74,* 33–41.

Gelles, R. J. (1987). *Family violence* (2nd ed.). Newbury Park, CA: Sage.

Gelman, D. (1989, January). The thoughts that wound. *Newsweek,* pp. 46–48.

Giacoletti, A. M. (1990). *Children's responses to parent and stranger dis-*

cord. Unpublished master's thesis, West Virginia University, Morgantown, WV.

Gjerde, P. F., Block, J. H., & Block, J. (1989). The family interaction Q-sort (FIQ). In H. D. Grotevant & C. I. Carlson (Eds.), *Handbook of family assessment*. New York: Guilford Press.

Glasberg, R., & Aboud, F. E. (1981). A developmental perspective on the study of depression: Children's evaluative reactions to sadness. *Developmental Psychology, 17,* 195–202.

Glasberg, R., & Aboud, F. E. (1982). Keeping one's distance from sadness: Children's self-reports of emotional experience. *Developmental Psychology, 18,* 287–293.

Glenn, N. D. (1987). Marriage on the rocks. *Psychology Today, 21,* 20–21.

Glenn, N. D. (1990). Quantitative research on marital quality in the 1980s: A critical review. *Journal of Marriage and the Family, 52,* 818–831.

Gotlib, I. H. (1992). Interpersonal and cognitive aspects of depression. *Current Directions in Psychological Science, 1,* 149–154.

Gottman, J. M. (1979). *Marital interaction: Experimental investigations.* New York: Academic Press.

Gottman, J. M., & Katz, L. F. (1989). Effects of marital discord on young children's peer interaction and health. *Developmental Psychology, 25,* 373–381.

Gottman, J. M., & Krokoff, L. J. (1989). Marital interaction and satisfaction: A longitudinal view. *Journal of Consulting and Clinical Psychology, 57,* 47–52.

Gottman, J. M., & Levenson, R. W. (1986). Assessing the role of emotion in marriage. *Behavioral Assessment, 8,* 31–48.

Gottman, J. M., Markman, H., & Notarius, C. (1977). The topography of marital conflict: A sequential analysis of verbal and nonverbal behavior. *Journal of Marriage and the Family, 39,* 461–477.

Gottman, J. M., & Porterfield, A. L. (1981). Communicative competence in the nonverbal behavior of married couples. *Journal of Marriage and the Family, 43,* 817–824.

Graham, P., Rutter, M., & George, S. (1973). Temperamental characteristics as predictors of behavior disorders in children. *American Journal of Orthopsychiatry, 43,* 328–339.

Greenberg, L., & Johnson, S. (1986). Emotionally focused couples therapy. In N. S. Jacobson & A. S. Gurman (Eds.), *Clinical handbook of marital therapy* (pp. 253–276). New York: Guilford Press.

Greenberg, L., & Johnson, S. (1988). *Emotionally focused therapy for couples*. New York: Guilford Press.

Greenberg, M. T., & Speltz, M. (1988). Attachment and the ontogeny of conduct problems. In J. Belsky & T. Nezworski (Eds.), *Clinical implications of attachment* (pp. 177–218). Hillsdale, NJ: Erlbaum.

Grossmann, K., Grossmann, K. E., Spangler, G., Suess, G., & Unzer, L. (1985). Maternal sensitivity and newborns' orientation responses as related to quality of attachment in Northern Germany. In I. Bretherton & E. Waters (Eds.), Growing points of attachment theory and research. *Monographs of the Society for Research in Child Development, 50* (1–2, Serial No. 209), 233–256.

Grych, J. H., & Fincham, F. D. (1990). Marital conflict and children's adjustment: A cognitive–contextual framework. *Psychological Bulletin, 108,* 267–290.

Grych, J. H., & Fincham, F. D. (1992). Interventions for children of divorce: Towards greater integration of research and action, *Psychological Bulletin, 111,* 434–454.

Grych, J. H., & Fincham, F. D. (1993). Children's appraisals of marital conflict: Initial investigations of the cognitive–contextual framework. *Child Development, 64,* 215–230.

Grych, J. H., Seid, M., & Fincham, F. D. (1991, April). Children's cognitive and affective responses to different forms of interparental conflict. In E. M. Cummings (Chair), *Children's responses to adults' conflicts and emotional expressions across contexts*. Symposium conducted at the meeting of the Society for Research in Child Development, Seattle, WA.

Grych, J. H., Seid, M., & Fincham, F. D. (1992). Assessing marital conflict from the child's perspective. *Child Development, 63,* 558–572.

Guerra, N. G., & Slaby, R. G. (1989). Evaluative factors in social problem solving by aggressive boys. *Journal of Abnormal Child Psychology, 17,* 277–289.

Guidubaldi, J., & Perry, J. D. (1985). Divorce and mental health sequelae for children: A two-year follow-up of a nationwide sample. *Journal of the American Academy of Child Psychiatry, 24,* 531–537.

Halford, W. K., & Sanders, M. R. (1990). The relationship between cognition and behavior during marital interaction. *Journal of Social and Clinical Psychology, 9,* 489–510.

Hammen, C. (1988). Self-cognitions, stressful events, and the prediction of depression in children of depressed mothers. *Journal of Abnormal Child Psychology, 16,* 347–367.

Hammen, C. (1992). Cognitive, life stress, and interpersonal approaches to a developmental psychopathology model of depression. *Development and Psychopathology, 4,* 189–206.

Hammen, C., Burge, D., & Stansbury, K. (1990). Relationship of mother and child variables to child outcomes in a high-risk sample: A causal modeling analysis. *Developmental Psychology, 26,* 24–30.

Harter, S. (1982). A cognitive–developmental approach to children's understanding of affect and trait labels. In F. C. Serafica (Ed.), *Social-cognitive development in context* (pp. 27–61). New York: Guilford Press.

Harter, S. (1983). Children's understanding of multiple emotions: A cognitive-developmental approach. In W. F. Overton (Ed.), *The relationship between social and cognitive development* (pp. 147–194). Hillsdale, NJ: Erlbaum.

Harter, S. (1985). Commentary on the need for a developmental perspective in understanding child and adolescent disorders. *Journal of Social and Clinical Psychology, 3,* 484–499.

Harter, S., Marold, D. B., & Whitesell, N. R. (1992). Model of psychosocial risk factors leading to suicidal ideation in young adolescents. *Development and Psychopathology, 4,* 167–188.

Hauser, S. T., Vieyra, M. A., Jacobson, A. M., & Wertlieb, D. (1985). Vulnerability and resilience in adolescence: Views from the family. *Journal of Early Adolescence, 5,* 81–100.

Hazan, C., & Shaver, P. R. (1990). Love and work: An attachment-theoretical perspective. *Journal of Personality and Social Psychology, 59,* 270–280.

Hennessy, K. D., Rabideau, G. J., Cicchetti, D., & Cummings, E. M. (in press). Responses of physically abused children to different forms of interadult anger. *Child Development.*

Herbert, T. B., Silver, R. C., & Ellard, J. H. (1991). Coping with an abusive relationship: I. How and why do women stay? *Journal of Marriage and the Family, 53,* 311–325.

Hershorn, M., & Rosenbaum, A. (1985). Children of marital violence:

A closer look at the unintended victims. *American Journal of Orthopsychiatry, 55,* 260–266.

Hess, R. D., & Camara, K. A. (1979). Post-divorce family relationships as mediating factors in consequences of divorce on children. *Journal of Social Issues, 35,* 79–96.

Hetherington, E. M. (1984). Stress and coping in children and families. In A. Doyle, D. Gold, & D. Moskowitz (Eds.), *Children in families under stress* (pp. 7–33). San Francisco: Jossey-Bass.

Hetherington, E. M. (1989). Coping with family transitions: Winners, losers, and survivors. *Child Development, 60,* 1–14.

Hetherington, E. M. (1993). Long-term outcomes of divorce and remarriage: The early adolescent years. In A. S. Masten (Chair), *Family processes and youth functioning during the early adolescent years.* Symposium conducted at the meeting of the Society for Research in Child Development, New Orleans, LA.

Hetherington, E. M., Clingempeel, W. G., Anderson, E. R., Deal, J. E., Hagan, M. S., Hollier, E. A., & Lindner, M. S. (1992). Coping with marital transitions. *Monographs of the Society for Research in Child Development, 57,* (1–2, Serial No. 227).

Hetherington, E. M., Cox, M., & Cox, R. (1976). Divorced fathers. *Family Coordinator, 25,* 417–428.

Hetherington, E. M., Cox, M., & Cox, R. (1982). Effects of divorce on parents and children. In M. Lamb (Ed.), *Nontraditional families* (pp. 233–288). Hillsdale, NJ: Erlbaum.

Hetherington, E. M., Cox, M., & Cox, R. (1985). Long-term effects of divorce and remarriage on the adjustment of children. *Journal of the American Academy of Child Psychiatry, 24,* 518–530.

Hetherington, E. M., & Martin, B. (1979). Family interaction. In H. C. Quay & J. S. Werry (Eds.), *Psychopathological disorders of childhood* (2nd ed., pp. 247–302). New York: Wiley.

Hill, J. P., Holmbeck, G. N., Marlow, L., Green, T. M., & Lynch, M. E. (1985). Pubertal status and parent–child relations in families of seventh-grade boys. *Journal of Early Adolescence, 5,* 31–44.

Hill, S. D., Bleichfeld, B., Brunstetter, R. D., Hebert, J. E., & Steckler, S. (1989). Cognitive and physiological responsiveness of abused children. *Journal of the American Academy of Child and Adolescent Psychiatry, 28,* 219–224.

Hoffman, M. A., Ushpiz, V., & Levy-Shiff, R. (1988). Social support and self-esteem in adolescence. *Journal of Youth and Adolescence, 17*, 307–316.

Holden, G. W., & Ritchie, K. L. (1991). Linking extreme marital discord, child rearing, and child behavior problems: Evidence from battered women. *Child Development, 62,* 311–327.

Holtzworth-Munroe, A. (1988). Causal attributions in marital violence: Theoretical and methodological issues. *Clinical Psychology Review, 8,* 331–344.

Holtzworth-Munroe, A., & Jacobson, N. S. (1985). Causal attributions of married couples: When do they search for causes? What do they conclude when they do? *Journal of Personality and Social Psychology, 48,* 1398–1412.

Hops, H., Biglan, A., Sherman, L., Arthur, J., Friedman, L., & Osteen, R. (1987). Home observations of family interactions of depressed women. *Journal of Consulting and Clinical Psychology, 55,* 341–346.

Hotaling, G. T., & Sugarman, D. B. (1990). A risk marker analysis of assaulted wives. *Journal of Family Violence, 5,* 1–13.

Howes, P., & Markman, H. J. (1989). Marital quality and child functioning: A longitudinal investigation. *Child Development, 60,* 1044–1051.

Hubbard, R. M., & Adams, C. F. (1936). Factors affecting the success of child guidance clinic treatment. *American Journal of Orthopsychiatry, 6,* 81–103.

Hughes, H. (1988). Psychological and behavioral correlates of family violence in child witnesses and victims. *American Journal of Orthopsychiatry, 58,* 77–90.

Hughes, H., Parkinson, D., & Vargo, M. (1989). Witnessing spouse abuse and experiencing physical abuse: A "double whammy"? *Journal of Family Violence, 4,* 197–209.

Ilfeld, F. W. (1980). Understanding marital stressors: The importance of coping style. *Journal of Nervous and Mental Disease, 168,* 375–381.

Isabella, R. A., & Belsky, J. (1985). Marital change during the transitions to parenthood and security of infant-parent attachment. *Journal of Family Issues, 6,* 505–522.

Izard, C. E., & Schwartz, G. M. (1986). Patterns of emotion in depression. In M. Rutter, C. E. Izard, & P. B. Read (Eds.), *Depression in young people: Developmental and clinical perspectives* (pp. 33–70). New York: Guilford Press.

Jacobson, D. S. (1978). The impact of marital separation/divorce on children: II. Interparent hostility and child adjustment. *Journal of Divorce, 2,* 3–19.

Jacobson, N. S. (1989). The politics of intimacy. *Behavior Therapist, 12,* 29–32.

Jacobson, N. S., Holtzworth-Munroe, A., & Schmaling, K. B. (1989). Marital therapy and spouse involvement in the treatment of depression, agoraphobia, and alcoholism. *Journal of Consulting and Clinical Psychology, 57,* 5–10.

Jacobson, N. S., & Margolin, G. (1979). *Marital therapy: Strategies based on social learning and behavior exchange principles.* New York: Brunner/Mazel.

Jacobson, N. S., & Moore, D. (1981). Spouses as observers of the events in their relationship. *Journal of Consulting and Clinical Psychology, 49,* 269–277.

Jaenicke, C., Hammen, C., Zupan, B., Hirito, D., Gordon, D., Adrian, C., & Burge, D. (1987). Cognitive vulnerability in children at risk for depression. *Journal of Abnormal Child Psychology, 15,* 559–572.

Jaffe, P., Wolfe, D., Wilson, S. K., & Zak, L. (1986). Family violence and child adjustment: A comparative analysis of girls' and boys' behavioral symptoms. *American Journal of Psychiatry, 143,* 74–77.

Jenkins, J. M., & Smith, M. A. (1991). Marital disharmony and children's behavior problems: Aspects of poor marriage that affect children adversely. *Journal of Child Psychology and Psychiatry, 32,* 793–810.

Johnson, P. L., & O'Leary, K. D. (1987). Parental behavior patterns and conduct disorders in girls. *Journal of Abnormal Child Psychology, 15,* 573–581.

Johnston, J. R., Gonzalez, R., & Campbell, L. E. (1987). Ongoing post-divorce conflict and child disturbance. *Journal of Abnormal Child Psychology, 15,* 497–509.

Jouriles, E. N., Barling, J., & O'Leary, K. D. (1987). Predicting child behavior problems in maritally violent families. *Journal of Abnormal Child Psychology, 15,* 165–173.

Jouriles, E. N., Bourg, W. J., & Farris, A. M. (1991). Marital adjustment and child conduct problems: A comparison of the correlation across subsamples. *Journal of Consulting and Clinical Psychology, 59,* 354–357.

Jouriles, E. N., Murphy, C. M., Farris, A. M., Smith, D. A., Richters, J. E., & Waters, E. (1991). Marital adjustment, parental disagreements about child rearing, and behavior problems in boys: Increasing the specificity of the marital assessment. *Child Development, 62,* 1424–1433.

Jouriles, E. N., Murphy, C. M., & O'Leary, K. D. (1989). Interspousal aggression, marital discord, and child problems. *Journal of Consulting and Clinical Psychology, 57,* 453–455.

Jouriles, E. N., Pfiffner, L. J., & O'Leary, S. G. (1988). Marital conflict, parenting, and toddler conduct problems. *Journal of Abnormal Child Psychology, 16,* 197–206.

Kaslow, H. J., Rehm, L. P., & Siegel, A. W. (1984). Social–cognitive and cognitive correlates of depression in children. *Journal of Abnormal Child Psychology, 12,* 605–620.

Keller, M. B., Beardslee, W. R., Dorer, D. J., Lavori, P. W., Samuelson, H., & Klerman, G. L. (1986). Impact of severity and chronicity of parental affective illness on adaptive functioning and psychopathology in children. *Archives of General Psychiatry, 43,* 930–937.

Klaczynski, P. A., & Cummings, E. M. (1989). Responding to anger in aggressive and nonaggressive boys. *Journal of Child Psychology and Psychiatry, 30,* 309–314.

Kline, M., Johnston, J. R., & Tschann, J. M. (1991). The long shadow of marital conflict: A model of children's postdivorce adjustment. *Journal of Marriage and the Family, 53,* 297–309.

Kobak, R., & Sceery, A. (1988). Attachment in later adolescence: Working models, affect regulation, and perceptions of self and others. *Child Development, 59,* 135–146.

Kobak, R., Sudler, N., & Gamble, W. (1991). Attachment and depressive symptoms during adolescence: A developmental pathways analysis. *Development and Psychopathology, 3,* 461–474.

Kopp, C. B. (1982). Antecedents of self-regulation: A developmental perspective. *Developmental Psychology, 18,* 199–214.

Kopp, C. B. (1989). Regulation of distress and negative emotions: A developmental view. *Developmental Psychology, 25,* 343–354.

Koren, P., Carlton, K., & Shaw, D. (1980). Marital conflict: Relations among behaviors, outcomes, and distress. *Journal of Consulting and Clinical Psychology, 48,* 460–468.

Kozak, M. J., & Miller, G. A. (1982). Hypothetical constructs versus intervening variables: A re-appraisal of the three-systems model of anxiety assessment. *Behavioral Assessment, 4,* 347–358.

Krokoff, L. J., Gottman, J. M., & Roy, A. K. (1988). Blue-collar and white-collar marital interaction and communication orientation. *Journal of Social and Personal Relationships, 5,* 201–221.

Kurdek, L. A. (1981). An integrative perspective on children's divorce adjustment. *American Psychologist, 36,* 856–866.

Kurdek, L. A. (1986). Children's reasoning about parental divorce. In R. D. Ashmore & D. M. Brodzinsky (Eds.), *Thinking about the family: Views of parents and children* (pp. 233–276). Hillsdale, NJ: Erlbaum.

Kyle, S. O., & Falbo, T. (1985). Relationships between marital stress and attributional preferences for own and spouse behavior. *Journal of Social and Clinical Psychology, 3,* 339–351.

Lamb, M. E. (1987). Predictive implications of individual differences in attachment. *Journal of Consulting and Clinical Psychology, 55,* 817–824.

Lang, P. J. (1968). Fear reduction and fear behavior: Problems in treating a construct. In J. M. Shlien (Ed.), *Research in psychotherapy* (Vol. 3, pp. 90–102). Washington, DC: American Psychological Association.

Lear, M. W. (1991, September). Staying together. *Ladies' Home Journal,* pp. 60–71.

Lee, C. L., & Bates, J. E. (1985). Mother-child interactions at two years and perceived difficult temperament. *Child Development, 56,* 1314–1325.

Levenson, R. W., & Gottman, J. M. (1983). Marital interaction: Physiological linkage and affective exchange. *Journal of Personality and Social Psychology, 45,* 587–597.

Levenson, R. W., & Gottman, J. M. (1985). Physiological and affective predictors of change in relationship satisfaction. *Journal of Personality and Social Psychology, 49,* 85–94.

Lewis, M., Feiring, C., McGuffog, C., & Jaskir, J. (1984). Predicting psychopathology in six-year-olds from early social relations. *Child Development, 55,* 123–136.

Lloyd, S. A. (1990). Conflict types and strategies in violent marriages. *Journal of Family Violence, 5,* 269–284.

Loeber, R., & Dishion, T. J. (1984). Boys who fight at home and school: Family conditions influencing cross-setting consistency. *Journal of Consulting and Clinical Psychology, 52,* 759–768.

Londerville, S., & Main, M. (1981). Security of attachment, compliance, and maternal training methods in the second year of life. *Developmental Psychology, 17,* 289–299.

Long, N., & Forehand, R. (1987). The effects of parental divorce and parental conflict on children: An overview. *Developmental and Behavioral Pediatrics, 8,* 292–296.

Long, N., Forehand, R., Fauber, R., & Brody, G. H. (1987). Self-perceived and independently observed competence of young adolescents as a function of parental marital conflict and recent divorce. *Journal of Abnormal Child Psychology, 15,* 15–27.

Long, N., Slater, E., Forehand, R., & Fauber, R. (1988). Continued high or reduced interparental conflict following divorce: Relation to young adolescent adjustment. *Journal of Consulting and Clinical Psychology, 56,* 467–469.

Lorber, R., Felton, D. K., & Reid, J. (1984). A social learning approach to the reduction of coercive processes in child abusive families: A molecular analysis. *Advances in Behavior Research and Therapy, 6,* 29–45.

Lytton, H. (1990). Child and parent effects in boys' conduct disorder: A reinterpretation. *Developmental Psychology, 26,* 683–697.

Lytton, J. (1991). Parents' differential socialization of boys and girls: A meta-analysis. *Psychological Bulletin, 109,* 267–296.

Maccoby, E., & Martin, J. (1983). Socialization in contexts of the family: Parent–child interaction. In E. M. Hetherington (Ed.), *Handbook of child psychology: Vol. 4. Socialization, personality, and social development* (4th ed., pp. 1–101). New York: Wiley.

Maccoby, E. E., Snow, M. E., & Jacklin, C. N. (1984). Children's dispositions and mother–child interaction at 12 and 18 months: A short-term longitudinal study. *Developmental Psychology, 20,* 459–472.

Madden, M. E., & Janoff-Bulman, R. (1981). Blame, control, and marital satisfaction: Wives' attributions for conflict in marriage. *Journal of Marriage and the Family, 43,* 663–674.

Main, M., & Cassidy, J. (1988). Catagories of response to reunion with the parent at age six: Predictable from infant attachment classifications and stable over a one-month period. *Developmental Psychology, 24,* 415–426.

Main, M., & Goldwyn, R. (1984). Predicting rejection of her infant from mother's representation of her own experiences: Implications for the abused–abusing intergenerational cycle. *Child Abuse and Neglect, 8,* 203–217.

Main, M., & Hesse, E. (1990). Parents' unresolved traumatic experiences are related to infant disorganized attachment status. In M. T. Greenberg, D. Cicchetti, & E. M. Cummings (Eds.), *Attachment in the preschool years: Theory, research, and intervention* (pp. 161–182). Chicago: University of Chicago Press.

Main, M., Kaplan, N., & Cassidy, J. (1985). Security in infancy, childhood, and adulthood: A move to the level of representation. In I. Bretherton & E. Waters (Eds.), Growing points of attachment research. *Monographs of the Society for Research in Child Development, 50* (1–2, Serial No. 209), 66–104.

Main, M., & Solomon, J. (1990). Procedures for identifying infants as disorganized/disoriented during the Ainsworth Strange Situation. In M. T. Greenberg, D. Cicchetti, & E. M. Cummings (Eds.), *Attachment in the preschool years: Theory, research, and intervention* (pp. 121–160). Chicago: University of Chicago Press.

Maiuro, R. D., Cahn, T. S., Vitaliano, P. P., Wagner, B., & Zegree, J. B. (1988). Anger, hostility, and depression in domestically violent versus generally assaultive men and nonviolent control subjects. *Journal of Consulting and Clinical Psychology, 56,* 17–23.

Mangelsdorf, S., Gunnar, M., Kestenbaum, R., Lang, S., & Andreas, D. (1990). Infant proneness-to-distress temperament, maternal personality, and mother–infant attachment: Associations and goodness of fit. *Child Development, 61,* 820–831.

Margolin, G. (1979). Conjoint marital therapy to enhance anger management and reduce spouse abuse. *American Journal of Family Therapy, 7,* 13–23.

Margolin, G., John, R., & Gleberman, L. (1988). Affective response to conflictual discussions in violent and nonviolent couples. *Journal of Consulting and Clinical Psychology, 56,* 24–33.

Margolin, G., John, R. S., & O'Brien, M. (1989). Home observations of married couples reenacting naturalistic conflicts. *Behavioral Assessment, 11,* 101–118.

Margolin, G., & Wampold, B. (1981). Sequential analysis of conflict and accord in distressed and nondistressed marital partners. *Journal of Consulting and Clinical Psychology, 49,* 554–567.

Margolin, G., & Weiss, R. L. (1978). Comparative evaluation of therapeutic components associated with behavioral marital treatments. *Journal of Consulting and Clinical Psychology, 46,* 1476–1486.

Markman, H. J., Duncan, S. W., Storaasli, R. D., & Howes, P. W. (1987). The prediction and prevention of marital distress: A longitudinal investigation. In K. Hahlweg & M. Goldstein (Eds.), *Understanding major mental disorders: The contribution of family interaction research* (pp. 266–289). New York: Family Process Press.

Markman, H. J., & Floyd, F. (1980). Possibilities for the prevention of marital discord: A behavioral perspective. *American Journal of Family Therapy, 8,* 29–48.

Markman, H. J., Floyd, F. J., Stanley, S. M., & Jamieson, K. (1984). A cognitive-behavioral program for the prevention of marital and family distress: Issues in program development and delivery. In K. Halweg & N. S. Jacobson (Eds.), *Marital interaction* (pp. 396–428). New York: Guilford Press.

Markman, H. J., Floyd, F. J., Stanley, S. M., & Lewis, H. C. (1986). Prevention. In N. S. Jacobson & A. S. Gurman (Eds.), *Clinical handbook of marital therapy* (pp. 173–195). New York: Guilford Press.

Markman, H. J., Floyd, F. J., Stanley, S. M., & Storaasli, R. D. (1988). Prevention of marital distress: A longitudinal investigation. *Journal of Consulting and Clinical Psychology, 56,* 210–217.

Markman, H. J., & Kraft, S. A. (1989). Men and women in marriage: Dealing with gender differences in marital therapy. *Behavior Therapist, 12,* 51–56.

Marvin, R. S., & Stewart, R. B. (1990). A family systems framework for the study of attachment. In M. Greenberg, D. Cicchetti, & E. M. Cummings (Eds.), *Attachment in the preschool years: Theory, research, and intervention* (pp. 51–86). Chicago: University of Chicago Press.

Mash, E. J., & Johnston, C. (1990). Determinants of parenting stress: Illustrations from families of hyperactive children and families of physically abused children. *Journal of Clinical Child Psychology, 19,* 313–328.

Medved, D. (1989). *The case against divorce.* New York: Donald I. Fine.

Menaghan, E. (1982). Measuring coping effectiveness: A panel analysis of marital problems and coping efforts. *Journal of Health and Social Behavior, 23,* 220–234.

Merikangas, K. R., Prusoff, B. A., Kupfer, D. J., & Frank, E. (1985).

Marital adjustment in depression. *Journal of Affective Disorders, 9,* 5–11.

Meyersberg, M. A., & Post, R. M. (1979). An holistic developmental view of neural and psychological processes: A neurobiological–psychoanalytic integration. *British Journal of Psychiatry, 135,* 139–155.

Miller, N. B., Cowan, P. A., Cowan, C. P., Hetherington, E. M., & Clingempeel, W. G. (1993). Externalizing in preschoolers and early adolescents: A cross-study replication of a family model. *Developmental Psychology, 29,* 3–18.

Minuchin, P. (1985). Families and individual development: Provocations from the field of family therapy. *Child Development, 56,* 289–302.

Montemayor, R. (1983). Parents and adolescents in conflict: All families some of the time and some families most of the time. *Journal of Early Adolescence, 3,* 83–103.

Mulaik, S. A. (1987). Toward a conception of causality applicable to experimentation and causal modeling. *Child Development, 58,* 18–32.

Myers, D. G. (1990). *Social psychology* (3rd ed.). New York: McGraw-Hill.

Newman, H. M., & Langer, E. J. (1988). Investigating the development and courses of intimate relationships. In L. Y. Abramson (Ed.), *Social cognition and clinical psychology: A synthesis* (pp. 148–173). New York: Guilford Press.

Niemi, P. M. (1988). Family interaction patterns and the development of social conceptions in the adolescent. *Journal of Youth and Adolescence, 17,* 429–444.

Nolen-Hoeksema, S. (1987). Sex differences in unipolar depression: Evidence and theory. *Psychological Bulletin, 101,* 259–282.

Noller, P. (1987). Nonverbal communication in marriage. In D. Perlman & S. Duck (Eds.), *Intimate relationships: Development, dynamics, and deterioration* (pp. 149–175). Newbury Park, CA: Sage.

Noller, P., & Fitzpatrick, M. A. (1990). Marital communication in the eighties. *Journal of Marriage and the Family, 52,* 832–843.

Notarius, C. I., Benson, P. R., Sloane, D., Vanzetti, N. A., Hornyak, L. M. (1989). Exploring the interface between perception and behavior: An analysis of marital interaction in distressed and nondistressed couples. *Behavioral Assessment, 11,* 39–64.

Notarius, C. I., & Johnson, J. S. (1982). Emotional expression in husbands and wives. *Journal of Marriage and the Family, 45,* 483–489.

O'Brien, M., Margolin, G., John, R. S., & Krueger, L. (1991). Mothers' and sons' cognitive and emotional reactions to simulated marital and family conflict. *Journal of Consulting and Clinical Psychology, 59,* 692–703.

O'Leary, K. D., & Smith, D. A. (1991). Marital interactions. *Annual Review of Psychology, 42,* 191–212.

Olweus, D. (1980). Familial and temperament determinants of aggressive behavior in adolescent boys: A causal analysis. *Developmental Psychology, 16,* 644–660.

Panak, W. F., & Garber, J. (1992). Role of aggression, rejection, and attributions in the prediction of depression in children. *Development and Psychopathology, 4,* 145–165.

Pastor, D. L. (1981). The quality of mother–infant attachment and its relationship to toddlers' initial sociability with peers. *Developmental Psychology, 17,* 326–335.

Patterson, G. R. (1980). Mothers: The unacknowledged victims. *Monographs of the Society for Research in Child Development, 45* (5, Serial No. 186).

Patterson, G. R. (1982). *Coercive family process.* Eugene, OR: Castalia Press.

Patterson, G. R. (1986). Performance models for antisocial boys. *American Psychologist, 41,* 432–444.

Patterson, G. R., Capaldi, D., & Bank, L. (1990). An early starter model for predicting delinquency. In D. Pepler & K. H. Rubin (Eds.), *The development and treatment of childhood aggression* (pp. 139–168). Hillsdale, NJ: Erlbaum.

Patterson, G. R., & Dishion, T. J. (1988). Multilevel family process models: Traits, interactions, and relationships. In R. Hinde & J. Stevenson-Hinde (Eds.), *Relationships within families: Mutual influences* (pp. 283–310). Oxford, England: Clarendon Press.

Pearlin, L. I., & Schooler, C. (1978). The structure of coping. *Journal of Health and Social Behavior, 19,* 2–21.

Pelham, W. E., Milich, R., Cummings, E. M., Murphy, D. A., Schaughency, E. A., & Greiner, A. R. (1991). Effects of background anger, provocation, and methylphenidate on emotional arousal and aggressive responding in attention-deficit hyperactivity disordered boys with and without concurrent aggressiveness. *Journal of Abnormal Child Psychology, 19,* 407–426.

Peterson, J. L., & Zill, N. (1986). Marital disruption, parent–child relationships, and behavior problems in children. *Journal of Marriage and the Family, 48,* 295–307.

Petit, G. S., & Bates, J. E. (1984). Continuity of individual differences in the mother-infant relationship from six to thirteen months. *Child Development, 55,* 729–739.

Petit, G. S., & Bates, J. E. (1989). Family interaction patterns and children's behavior problems from infancy to 4 years. *Developmental Psychology, 25,* 413–420.

Petit, G. S., & Dodge, K. A., & Brown, M. M. (1988). Early family experience, social problem solving patterns, and children's social competence. *Child Development, 59,* 107–120.

Plomin, R. (1989). Environment and genes: Determinants of behavior. *American Psychologist, 44,* 105–111.

Porter, B., & O'Leary, K. D. (1980). Marital discord and childhood behavior problems. *Journal of Abnormal Child Psychology, 8,* 287–295.

Pruitt, D. G., & Rubin, J. Z. (1986). *Social Conflict: Escalation, stalemate, and settlement.* New York: Random House.

Radke-Yarrow, M., Cummings, E. M., Kuczynski, L., & Chapman, M. (1985). Patterns of attachment in two- and three-year-olds in normal families and families with parental depression. *Child Development, 56,* 884–893.

Radke-Yarrow, M., Zahn-Waxler, C., & Chapman, M. (1983). Children's prosocial dispositions and behavior. In E. M. Hetherington (Ed.), *Handbook of child psychology: Socialization, personality, and social development* (4th ed., pp. 469–546). New York: Wiley.

Reichenbach, L., & Masters, J. C. (1983). Children's use of expressive and contextual cues in judgments of emotion. *Child Development, 54,* 993–1004.

Reiss, D., Plomin, R., & Hetherington, E. M. (1991). Genetics and psychiatry: An unheralded window on the environment. *American Journal of Psychiatry, 148,* 283–291.

Robins, L. N. (1966). *Deviant children grown up.* Baltimore: Williams & Wilkins.

Robinson, E., & Price, M. G. (1980). Pleasurable behavior in marital interaction: An observational study. *Journal of Consulting and Clinical Psychology, 48,* 117–118.

Rose, D., & Abramson, L. Y. (1992). Developmental predictors of depressive cognitive style: Research and theory. In D. Cicchetti & S. Toth (Eds.), *Rochester Symposium on Developmental Psychopathology: Vol. 4. Developmental approaches to depression* (pp. 323–349). Rochester, NY: University of Rochester Press.

Rosen, M. D., Moschetta, E. F., & Moschetta, P. (1991, December). Can this marriage be saved? A workbook for you and your husband. *Ladies' Home Journal*, pp. 69–73.

Rosenbaum, A., & O'Leary, K. D. (1981). Marital violence: Characteristics of abusive couples. *Journal of Consulting and Clinical Psychology, 49,* 63–71.

Rosenbaum, A., & O'Leary, K. D. (1986). The treatment of marital violence. In N. S. Jacobson & A. S. Gurman (Eds.), *Clinical handbook of marital therapy* (pp. 385–405). New York: Guilford Press.

Rossman, B. B. R., & Rosenberg, M. S. (1992). Family stress and functioning in children: The moderating effects of children's beliefs about their control over parental conflict. *Journal of Child Psychology and Psychiatry, 33,* 699–715.

Rubin, K. H., & Lollis, S. P. (1988). Origins and consequences of social withdrawal. In J. Belsky & T. Nezworski (Eds.), *Clinical implications of attachment* (pp. 219–252). Hillsdale, NJ: Erlbaum.

Rutter, M. (1970). Sex differences in response to family stress. In E. J. Anthony & C. Koupernik (Eds.), *The child in his family* (pp. 165–196). New York: Wiley.

Rutter, M. (1971). Parent–child separation: Psychological effects on children. *Journal of Child Psychology and Psychiatry, 12,* 233–260.

Rutter, M. (1979). Maternal deprivation, 1972–1978: New findings, new concepts, new approaches. *Child Development, 50,* 283–305.

Rutter, M. (1980). *Changing youth in a changing society.* Cambridge, MA: Harvard University Press.

Rutter, M. (1981). Stress, coping, and development: Some issues and some questions. *Journal of Child Psychology and Psychiatry,* 323–356.

Rutter, M. (1986). The developmental psychopathology of depression: Issues and perspectives. In M. Rutter, C. E. Izard, & P. B. Read (Eds.), *Depression in young people: Developmental and clinical perspectives* (pp. 3–30). New York: Guilford Press.

Rutter, M. (1990a). Psychosocial resilience and protective mechanisms. In J. Rolf, A. S. Masten, D. Cicchetti, K. H. Neuchterlein, & S. Weintraub (Eds.), *Risk and protective factors in the development of psychopathology* (pp. 181–214). Cambridge, England: Cambridge University Press.

Rutter, M. (1990b). Commentary: Some focus and process considerations regarding the effects of parental depression on children. *Developmental Psychology, 26,* 60–67.

Rutter, M., & Quinton, D. (1984). Parental psychiatric disorder: Effects on children. *Psychological Medicine, 14,* 853–880.

Rutter, M., Yule, B., Quinton, D., Rowlands, O., Yule, W., & Berger, M. (1974). Attainment and adjustment in two geographical areas: III. Some factors accounting for area differences. *British Journal of Psychiatry, 125,* 520–533.

Schneider-Rosen, K., & Cicchetti, D. (1984). The relationship between affect and cognition in maltreated infants: Quality of attachment and the development of visual self-recognition. *Child Development, 55,* 648–658.

Schwarz, J. C. (1979). Childhood origins of psychopathology. *American Psychologist, 34,* 879–885.

Sears, R. R., Maccoby, E. E., & Levine, H. (1957). *Patterns of child rearing.* Evanston, IL: Row-Peterson.

Selman, R. L. (1980). *The growth of interpersonal understanding: Developmental and clinical analyses.* New York: Academic Press.

Shaw, D. S., & Emery, R. E. (1987). Parental conflict and other correlates of adjustment in school-age children whose parents have separated. *Journal of Abnormal Child Psychology, 15,* 269–281.

Shaw, D. S., & Emery, R. E. (1988). Chronic family adversity and school-age children's adjustment. *Journal of the American Academy of Child and Adolescent Psychiatry, 27,* 200–206.

Shred, R., McDonnell, P. M., Church, G., & Rowan, J. (1991, April). *Infants' cognitive and emotional responses to adults' angry behavior.* Paper presented at the biennial meeting of the Society for Research in Child Development, Seattle, WA.

Simpson, K. S., & Cummings, E. M. (1993). *Verbal and nonverbal affective consistency of conflict resolution and children's responses to interadult anger.* Unpublished manuscript, West Virginia University, Morgantown, WV.

Slater, E. J., & Haber, J. D. (1984). Adolescent adjustment following divorce as a function of familial conflict. *Journal of Consulting and Clinical Psychology, 52,* 920–921.

Smith, D. A., Vivian, D., & O'Leary, K. D. (1990). Longitudinal prediction of marital discord from premarital expressions of affect. *Journal of Consulting and Clinical Psychology, 58,* 790–798.

Smolowe, J. (1991, January). Can't we talk this over? *Time,* p. 77.

Snyder, D. K., Klein, M. A., Gdowski, C. L., Faulstich, C., & La-Combe, J. (1988). Generalized dysfunction in clinic and non-clinic families: A comparative analysis. *Journal of Abnormal Child Psychology, 16,* 97–109.

Speltz, M. L. (1990). The treatment of preschool conduct problems. In M. T. Greenberg, D. Cicchetti, & E. M. Cummings (Eds.), *Attachment in the preschool years: Theory, research, and intervention* (pp. 399–426). Chicago: University of Chicago Press.

Speltz, M. L., Greenberg, M. T., & Dyklyen, M. (1990). Attachment in preschoolers with disruptive behavior: A comparison of clinic-referred and nonproblem children. *Development and Psychopathology, 2,* 31–46.

Sroufe, L. A. (1983). Infant–caregiver attachment and patterns of adaptation in preschool: The roots of maladaptation and competence. In M. Perlmutter (Ed.), *Minnesota Symposium in Child Psychology* (vol. 16, pp. 41–81). Hillsdale, NJ: Erlbaum.

Sroufe, L. A. (1985). Attachment classification from the perspective of infant–caregiver relationships and infant temperament. *Child Development, 56,* 1–14.

Sroufe, L. A. (1988). The role of infant–caregiver attachment in development. In J. Belsky & T. Nezworski (Eds.), *Clinical implications of attachment* (pp. 18–38). Hillsdale, NJ: Erlbaum.

Sroufe, L. A., & Fleeson, J. (1986). Attachment and the construction of relationships. In W. Hartup & Z. Rubin (Eds.), *Relationships and development* (pp. 51–71). Hillsdale, NJ: Erlbaum.

Sroufe, L. A., Fox, N. E., & Pancake, V. R. (1983). Attachment and dependency in developmental perspective. *Child Development, 54,* 1615–1627.

Sroufe, L. A., & Rutter, M. (1984). The domain of developmental psychopathology. *Child Development, 55,* 17–29.

Sroufe, L. A., & Waters, E. (1977). Attachment as an organizational construct. *Child Development, 48,* 1184–1199.

Steger, C., & Kotler, T. (1979). Contrasting resources in disturbed and non-disturbed family systems. *British Journal of Medical Psychology, 52,* 243–251.

Steinfeld, G. J. (1986). Spouse abuse: Clinical implications of research on the control of aggression. *Journal of Family Violence, 1,* 197–208.

Sternberg, K. J., Lamb, M. E., Greenbaum, C., Cicchetti, D., Dawud, S., Cortes, R. M., Krispin, O., & Lorey, F. (1993). Effects of domestic violence on children's behavior problems and depression. *Developmental Psychology, 29,* 44–52.

Stevenson-Hinde, J. (1990). Attachment within the family system: An overview. *Infant Mental Health Journal, 11,* 218–227.

Straus, M. A., Gelles, R., & Steinmetz, S. (1980). *Behind closed doors: Violence in the American family.* New York: Anchor Press.

Thompson, R. A. (1986). Temperament, emotionality, and infant social cognition. In J. V. Lerner & R. M. Lerner (Eds.), *Temperament and social interaction in infants and children* (pp. 35–52). San Francisco: Jossey-Bass.

Toth, S. L., Manly, J. T., & Cicchetti, D. (1992). Child maltreatment and vulnerability to depression. *Development and Psychopathology, 4,* 97–112.

Towle, C. (1931). The evaluation and management of marital status in foster homes. *American Journal of Orthopsychiatry, 1,* 271–284.

Trickett, P. K., Aber, J. L., Carlson, V., & Cicchetti, D. (1991). Relationship of socioeconomic status to the etiology and developmental sequelae of physical child abuse. *Developmental Psychology, 27,* 148–158.

Trickett, P. K., & Susman, E. J. (1989). Perceived similarities and disagreements about child-rearing practices in abusive and nonabusive families: Intergenerational and concurrent family processes. In D. Cicchetti & V. Carlson (Eds.), *Child maltreatment: Theory and research on the causes and consequences of child abuse and neglect* (pp. 280–301). New York: Cambridge University Press.

Tronick, E. Z. (1989). Emotions and emotional communication in infants. *American Psychologist, 44,* 112–119.

Tschann, J. M., Johnston, J. R., Kline, M., & Wallerstein, J. S. (1989). Family process and children's functioning during divorce. *Journal of Marriage and the Family, 51,* 431–444.

U. S. Bureau of the Census (1985). *Current Population Reports,* Series P-23, No. 141. Child support and alimony: 1983. Washington, DC: U. S. Government Printing Office.

Vasta, R. (1982). Physical child abuse: A dual-component analysis. *Developmental Review, 2,* 125–149.

Vaughn, B. E., Stevenson-Hinde, J., Waters, E., Kotsaftis, A., Lefever, G. B., Shouldice, A., Trudel, M., & Belsky, J. (1992). Attachment security and temperament in infancy and early childhood: Some conceptual clarifications. *Developmental Psychology, 28,* 463–473.

Vuchinich, S., Emery, R. E., & Cassidy, J. (1988). Family members as third parties in dyadic family conflict: Strategies, alliances, and outcomes. *Child Development, 59,* 1293–1302.

Walker, E., Downey, G., & Nightingale, N. (1989). The nonorthogonal nature of risk factors: Implications for research on the causes of maladjustment. *Journal of Primary Prevention, 9,* 143–163.

Wallace, R. (1935). A study of relationship between emotional tone in the home and adjustment status in cases referred to a traveling child guidance clinic. *Journal of Juvenile Research, 19,* 205–220.

Wallerstein, J. S. (1985). Children of divorce: Preliminary report of ten-year follow-up study of older children and adolescents. *Journal of the American Academy of Child Psychiatry, 24,* 545–553.

Wallerstein, J. S., & Blakeslee, S. (1989). *Second chances: Men, women, and children a decade after divorce.* New York: Ticknor & Fields.

Wallerstein, J. S., & Kelly, J. (1980). *Surviving the breakup: How children and parents cope with divorce.* New York: Basic Books.

Waters, E. (1978). The reliability and stability of individual differences in infant–mother attachment. *Child Development, 49,* 483–494.

Watson, J. B. (1925). *Behaviorism.* New York: W. W. Norton.

Webster-Stratton, C. (1981). Videotape modeling: A method of parent education. *Journal of Clinical Child Psychology, 10,* 93–97.

Webster-Stratton, C. (1990). Stress: A disruptor of parent perceptions and family interactions. *Journal of Clinical Child Psychology, 19,* 302–312.

Webster-Stratton, C., & Hammond, M. (1988). Maternal depression and its relationship to life stress, perceptions of child behavior problems, parenting behaviors, and child conduct problems. *Journal of Abnormal Child Psychology, 16,* 299–315.

Webster-Stratton, C., Hollinsworth, T., & Kolpacoff, M. (1989). The long-term effectiveness and clinical significance of three cost-effective training programs for families with conduct-problem children. *Journal of Consulting and Clinical Psychology, 57,* 550–553.

Webster-Stratton, C., Kolpacoff, M., & Hollinsworth, T. (1988). Self-administered videotape therapy for families with conduct-problem children: Comparison with two cost-effective treatments and a control group. *Journal of Consulting and Clinical Psychology, 56,* 558–566.

Welch, C. E., & Price-Bonham, S. (1983). A decade of no-fault divorce revisited: California, Georgia, and Washington. *Journal of Marriage and the Family, 45,* 411–418.

Werner, E. E. (1989). High-risk children in young adulthood: A longitudinal study from birth to 32 years. *American Journal of Orthopsychiatry, 59,* 72–81.

West, D. J., & Farrington, D. P. (1973). *Who becomes delinquent? A second report of the Cambridge study in delinquent development.* London: Heinemann.

West, M. O., & Prinz, R. J. (1987). Parental alcoholism and childhood psychopathology. *Psychological Bulletin, 102,* 204–218.

Whiffen, V. E., & Gotlib, I. H. (1989). Stress and coping in maritally distressed and nondistressed couples. *Journal of Social and Personal Relationships, 6,* 327–344.

Whitehead, B. F. (1993, April). Dan Quayle was right. *The Atlantic,* pp. 47–84.

Whitehead, L. (1979). Sex differences in children's responses to family stress. *Journal of Child Psychology and Psychiatry, 20,* 247–254.

Wierson, M., Forehand, R., & McCombs, A. (1988). The relationship of early adolescent functioning to parent-reported and adolescent-perceived interparental conflict. *Journal of Abnormal Child Psychology, 16,* 707–718.

Wolfe, D. A. (1985). Child-abusive parents: An empirical review and analysis. *Psychological Bulletin, 97,* 462–482.

Wolfe, D. A. (1987). *Child abuse: Implications for child development and psychopathology.* Beverly Hills, CA: Sage.

Wolfe, D. A., Jaffe, P., Wilson, S. K., & Zak, L. (1985). Children of battered women: The relation of child behavior to family violence and maternal stress. *Journal of Consulting and Clinical Psychology, 53,* 657–665.

Zahn-Waxler, C., Cummings, E. M., McKnew, D. H., & Radke-Yarrow, M. (1984). Altrusim, aggression, and social interactions in young children with a manic–depressive parent. *Child Development, 55,* 112–122.

Zahn-Waxler, C., Iannotti, R. J., Cummings, E. M., & Denham, S.

(1990). Antecedents of problem behaviors in children of depressed mothers. *Development and Psychopathology, 2,* 271–291.

Zahn-Waxler, C., Kochanska, G., Krupnick, J., & McKnew, D. (1990). Antecedents of problem behaviors in children of depressed mothers. *Developmental Psychology, 26,* 51–59.

Zahn-Waxler, C., Radke-Yarrow, M., & King, R. A. (1979). Child rearing and children's prosocial initiations toward victims of distress. *Child Development, 50,* 319–330.

Zaslow, M. J. (1988). Sex differences in children's response to parental divorce: 1. Research methodology and postdivorce family form. *American Journal of Orthopsychiatry, 58,* 355–378.

Zaslow, M. J. (1989). Sex differences in children's response to parental divorce: 2. Samples, variables, ages, and sources. *American Journal of Orthopsychiatry, 59,* 118–141.

Zaslow, M. J., & Hayes, C. D. (1986). Sex differences in children's response to psychosocial stress: Toward a cross-context analysis. In M. E. Lamb, A. L. Bron, & B. Rogoff (Eds.), *Advances in developmental psychology* (Vol. 4, pp. 285–337). Hillsdale, NJ: Erlbaum.

Zeanah, C. H., & Zeanah, P. D. (1989). Intergenerational transmission of maltreatment: Insights from attachment theory and research. *Psychiatry, 52,* 177–196.

Zigler, E., & Hall, N. W. (1989). Physical child abuse in America: Past, present, & future. In D. Cicchetti & S. Toth (Eds.), *Child maltreatment: Theory and research on the causes and consequences of child abuse and neglect* (pp. 38–75). Cambridge, England: Cambridge University Press.

Zillmann, D. (1971). Excitation transfer in communicated aggressive behavior. *Journal of Experimental Social Psychology, 7,* 419–434.

Zillmann, D. (1982). Cognitive and affective influences: Television viewing and arousal. In *Television and behavior: Ten years of scientific progress and implications for the 1980s: Vol. 2. Technical reviews.* Washington, DC: U. S. Government Printing Office.

Zillmann, D. (1983). Arousal and aggression. In R. G. Geen & E. I. Donnerstein (Eds.), *Aggression: Theoretical and empirical reviews: Vol. 1. Theoretical and methodological issues* (pp. 75–101). New York: Academic Press.

Index

Abuse
  of children, 7–8
    and responses of child to
      anger, 47, 83
    spousal, 18
      witnessed by children, 8,
      66–67
Academic performance of chil-
    dren from high-conflict
    homes, 5
Age of children
  and changes in response pat-
    terns, 119
  and developmental patterns,
    127–129
  and responses to interadult
    conflict, 58–59, 101–102,
    140–141
Aggression
  caused by parental emotional
    rejection of child, 95
  in children exposed to mari-
    tal anger, 4, 45–47, 83–
    84, 137
    conflict resolution affecting,
    70

as maladaptive coping pat-
    tern, 90
  modeling processes in, 46,
    93
  interspousal, responses of
    children to, 66–67, 81
  parental, toward children, 7–
    8
Alcoholic parents, children of,
    84–85
Alienation. *See* Withdrawal
Anger
  in depressed parents, 6–7
  in distressed marriages, 2,
    14–15
    responses of children to,
    40–61. *See also* Children's
    responses to interadult
    conflict
  laboratory simulation of, re-
    sponses to, 49–50
  nonverbal, 142–143
    assessing impact of, 112–
    113
    responses of children to,
    67–68, 83